Feed
Yourself,
Feed
Your
Family

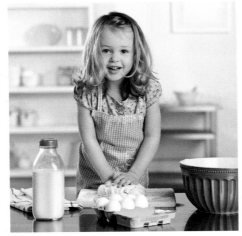

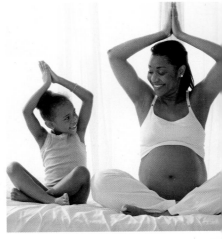

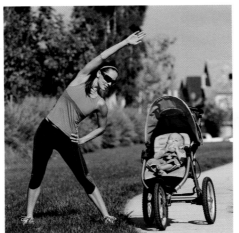

Good Nutrition
and Healthy
Cooking
for New Moms
and Growing
Families

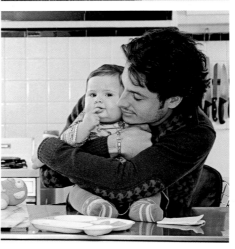

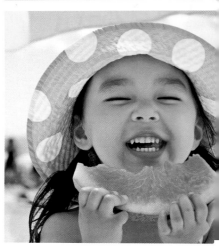

BALLANTINE BOOKS TRADE PAPERBACKS NEW YORK

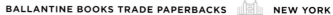

Feed Yourself, Feed Your Family

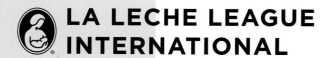

LA LECHE LEAGUE
INTERNATIONAL

No book can replace the diagnostic expertise and medical advice of a trusted physician. Please be certain to consult with your doctor before making any decisions that affect your health, particularly if you suffer from any medical condition or have any symptom that may require treatment.

As of press time, the URLs displayed in this book link or refer to existing websites on the Internet. Random House, Inc., is not responsible for, and should not be deemed to endorse or recommend, any website other than its own, or any content available on the Internet (including without limitation at any website, blog page, information page) that is not created by Random House.

A Ballantine Books Trade Paperback Original

Copyright © 2012 by La Leche League International

Published in the United States by Ballantine Books, an imprint of
The Random House Publishing Group, a division of Random House, Inc., New York.

BALLANTINE and colophon are registered trademarks of Random House, Inc.

Photo credits are located beginning on page 265.

Library of Congress Cataloging-in-Publication Data

Feed yourself, feed your family : good nutrition and healthy cooking for new moms and growing families / La Leche League International.
    p. cm.
Includes bibliographical references and index.
ISBN 978-0-345-51846-0 (pbk. : alk. paper) — ISBN 978-0-440-42365-2 (ebook)
1. Cooking (Natural foods) 2. Children—Nutrition. 3. Newborn infants—Nutrition.
4. Cooking, American. 5. Motherhood. I. La Leche League International.
TX741.F44 2012
641.3'02—dc23   2011044919

Printed in the United States of America

www.ballantinebooks.com

9 8 7 6 5 4 3 2 1

Book design by Liz Cosgrove

This book is dedicated to all the families who strive daily to make healthy choices in all parts of their lives—they know a loving enviroment is just as important to your family as what you eat.

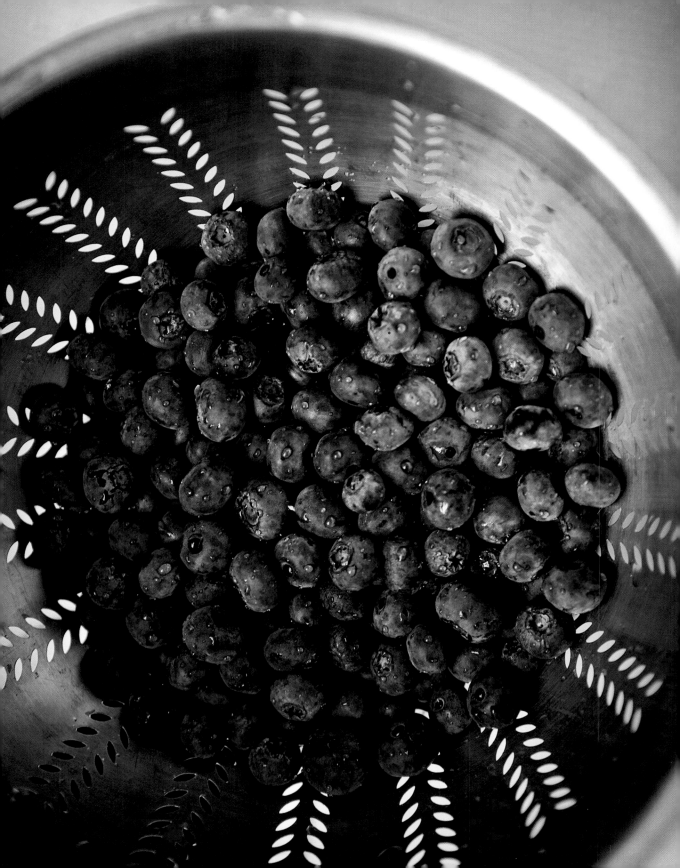

Contents

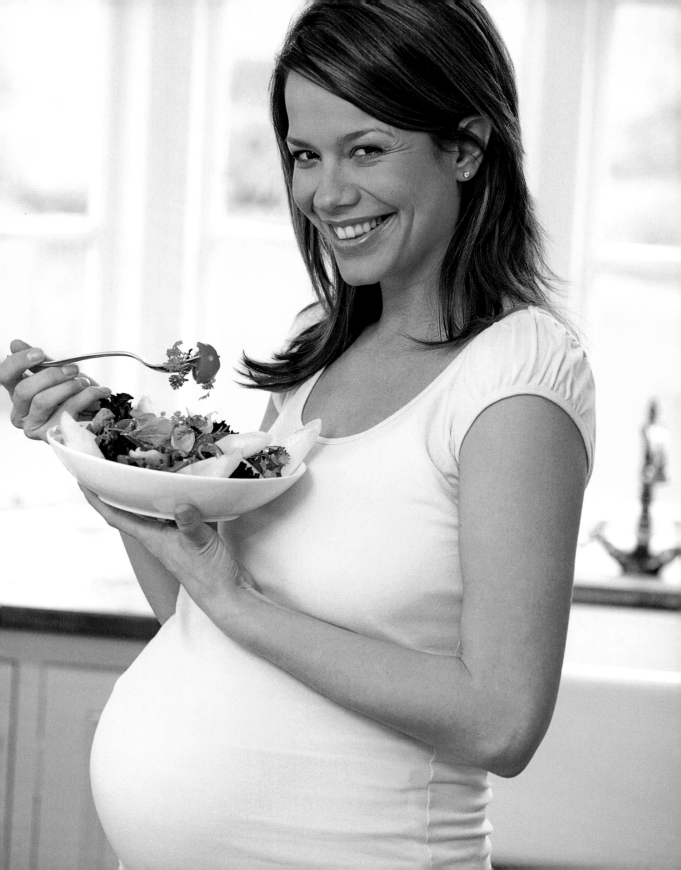

Introduction

What's Good for You Is Good for Your Family

When you had just one appetite to satisfy (yours), heeding the I-need-something-to-eat call was fairly simple.

Assuming you took the usual approach, you aimed for three meals a day, snacked here and there, and didn't stress too much about a late lunch, your growling stomach, your partner bringing home take-out Chinese (again), or having nothing in the fridge but a foil packet of ketchup and an apple or two. If your energy dipped at work, perhaps you grabbed coffee (and a handful of chocolates from a colleague's candy dish) and powered through to dinnertime without a snack. Maybe you were the type to let your cupboards run bare like Old Mother Hubbard before you dragged yourself to the store, since you ate most meals out. Maybe you were a foodie who enjoyed showing off occasionally at the stove. Or maybe you were somewhere in between, with most staples on hand and a few reliable recipes up your sleeve. In short, whether you were an ordinary eater or an all-out gourmet, you probably didn't plan your whole life around what and when you ate.

And then, one day, you weren't feeding just one person.

• • •

When you are pregnant and after your baby arrives, old patterns such as skipping breakfast, lunching on the daily fast-food special, going hungry for long stretches at a time, or eating a heavy, late-night dinner can carry consequences. Just to be clear, the consequences are for **you**—even if you subsist on chips and salsa, your growing baby will extract whatever essential nutrients she needs from your body to stay healthy, and she'll usually do just fine; you, on the other hand, may feel pretty crummy, whether it's low energy or an upset stomach.* Even if you consider yourself to be a fairly healthful eater and you score low on bad habits, motherhood—from pregnancy through nursing and beyond—can upend your approach to food and hunger, and your virtuous eating style can go right out the window, along with the pants that no longer fit.

If you're pregnant right now, you already know that eating takes on a new dimension when you have more than your own needs at stake. If you're currently nursing, the same holds true: you're feeding another body now. And if you have a nursling **and** other hungry folks both large and small in your household who look to you when they get hungry, your responsibilities will weigh even more heavily. Even if you have a helpful partner or older child who can help in the kitchen, you may be feeling that your "motherload" is harder to carry than a napping baby and an overloaded diaper bag.

But there's no need for guilt, anxiety, or whatever other stressful emotions mealtime may set off in your household. We think there has been way too much of that over the years when it comes to food and eating—**and** being a mother. Now that you've gone from "me" to "family," don't set a place at the table for guilt and its cousins. Instead, we want you to replace it with pleasure: the pleasure of preparing and eating good food for yourself and others, of feeding the ones you love, of joining together to nourish and nurture one another. That's what **Feed Yourself, Feed Your Family** is all about.

At La Leche League International (LLLI), our mission is to help mothers worldwide to breastfeed through mother-to-mother support, encouragement, information, and education, and to promote breastfeeding as an important ele-

---

* During pregnancy a baby takes nutrients from the mother, but if the mother isn't eating enough (that is, if she truly does subsist on a diet of chips and salsa), she may have inadequate weight gain and could deliver a low-birth-weight baby, who in turn could be at risk for serious illness.

ment in the healthy development of the baby and mother. So how does eating figure into our mission? We think there's a direct link: whether or not you're new to breastfeeding, you're more likely to be successful at it if you take care of yourself by eating well. That includes meeting your nutritional needs as well as your child's at various stages of motherhood, **and** your desire for good-tasting, healthful, simple-to-prepare food, from snacks to breakfasts, lunches, and dinners (and dessert, too).

If you eat well, your family will, too. Your growing baby's nutritional needs are met beautifully by breastfeeding. For older kids and other adults in your household, your commitment to taking care of yourself by eating properly will translate into satisfying family meals or meals for one or two, healthy snacks, quick and easy lunches, special-occasion foods, and treats, as well as a well-stocked kitchen, refrigerator, and pantry. With the appealing and adaptable recipes, nutritional information, and practical tips you'll find in the pages that follow, you won't scramble at mealtimes or have to head to the grocery store more than you want to. No more cupboard running bare—the only thing you and Old Mother Hubbard will have in common is that you're both moms!

How to Get the Most Out of This Book

We've organized **Feed Yourself, Feed Your Family** into chapters that correspond to your transition into motherhood, beginning with pregnancy. In each chapter, we'll discuss how good nutrition and a positive relationship with food support successful breastfeeding. You'll find nutritional information for whatever stage of motherhood you happen to be in, ideas for snacks and meals that you can make for yourself or for your growing family, and a selection of recipes at the end of each chapter. For instance:

- **If you're pregnant:** You'll want foods that will get you to the finish line feeling strong and ready for breastfeeding. See the nutritional info and snack and meal ideas in Chapter 1 and try out the recipes at the end of each chapter, rich in vital nutrients like iron, calcium, and folate: Veggie and Beef

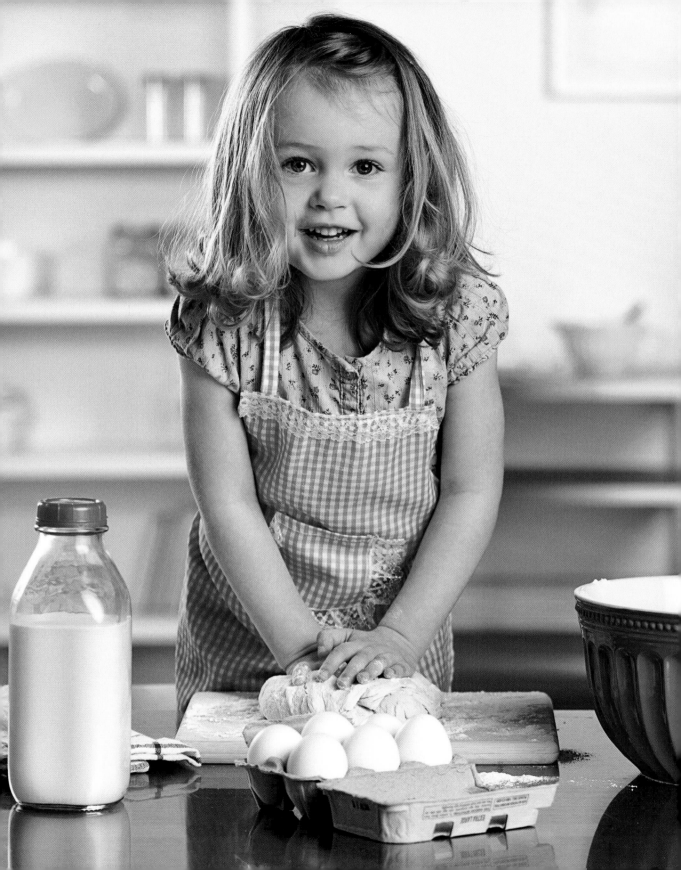

Meatloaf (page 176), Sautéed Spinach with Garlic (page 51), Calico Bean Salad (page 54), and many more.

- **If you have a newborn:** Try the easy-to-prepare foods you can eat with one hand on pages 65–66—because you're using your other one to hang on to your nursling! If you've got a friend or relative who'd love to bring you a meal, suggest our hearty, classic (and freezer-friendly) Three-Cheese Lasagna with Italian Sausage, on page 81, which has satisfied generations of new moms. Get your calcium with our delicious Super Smoothie with Yogurt, Berries, and Bananas recipe on page 103.

- **If you're back at work after maternity leave,** managing an overflowing in-box and a little night owl who wants a late-night or early-morning meal, you need quick and easy recipes all day long. When you're out the door and on the go, an Apple Bran Muffin (recipe on page 146) is a healthy way to start your workday or break for an afternoon snack. You'll also appreciate how many of our recipes can be made ahead, prepared in a slow cooker, prepped in under 30 minutes, or frozen—smart dinner solutions for busy weeknights.

- **If you've got more than one hungry diner to feed:** Experiment with recipes such as Red Onion and Olive Roasted Chicken Pieces (page 130), which can be adapted for grown-up tastes and kids' palates (turn up the flavor with the onions and olives, or set aside a milder version for your younger eaters), a convenient one-dish oven dinner that gives you more time for mothering. When your newest family member is ready to join you at the table, you'll be ready with the ideas, information, and recipes you'll find in Chapters 4 and 5.

- **If you want some help along the way:** Learn how to turn offers of "Can I help?" into plates of food with recipes such as our freezer-friendly Turkey Shepherd's Pie with Sweet Potatoes (page 42). When friends from work or family members call and ask, "What do you need?" say, "Dinner!" and ask them to make two pies—one for now and one for next week! If your partner and other children, if you have them, want to roll up their sleeves and get cooking, send them into the kitchen with family favorites such as Homemade Mac and Cheese (page 231), Broccoli with Parmesan Crumbs (page 96), and One-Bowl Chocolate Cake (page 240).

Here are well-balanced and nutritious main dishes that will satisfy you and your family, plus healthy sides and guilt-free treats. Don't hesitate to skip around and read whatever chapter appeals to you. Though we have arranged chapters and nutritional information in chronological order that makes sense for new moms, a recipe or snack idea in the middle or at the end of the book may well interest you or trigger your taste buds. Throughout this book you'll see some honest comments and mother-to-mother tips from the many visitors to our popular forums on the LLLI website. All of these women are breastfeeding moms at different stages—just like you.

About the Recipes

More than a dozen of the recipes in **Feed Yourself, Feed Your Family** are longtime favorites submitted by members of La Leche League—actually, by several generations of members! (In some cases, older recipes have been updated or revised to reflect today's ingredients and cooking techniques.) Recipes such as the Greek-flavored soup Avgolemono, classic Banana-Nut Bread, and our reliable La Leche League Baking Mix (for pancakes, waffles, and quick breads) have hit the spot for countless hungry La Leche League families, and we're including these Member's Favorite recipes here because they are classics that still satisfy.

If you are using nonstick cookware, you may be able to cut back on the amount of oil used to sauté or stir-fry various ingredients. Many recipes call for two or more tablespoons of oil, but you can often coat the bottom of a nonstick pan with half that amount. Experiment with what works best in your kitchen. If you are concerned about reducing fat in dishes containing items such as sour cream, milk, cheese, and butter, consider using less than the amount specified, or try substituting lower-fat varieties. Please note that the recipes have all been tested with the amounts and types of fats and oils specified in the ingredient listings.

LOOK FOR THESE SYMBOLS BY SELECT RECIPES YOU'LL FIND AT THE END OF EACH CHAPTER:

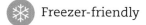 Quick—active prep time is under 30 minutes

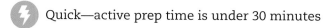 Freezer-friendly

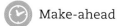 Make-ahead

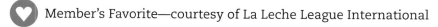 Member's Favorite—courtesy of La Leche League International

Perhaps you have seen some of our members' other oldies-but-goodies in one of the now-classic cookbooks published by La Leche League International, such as **Whole Foods for the Whole Family** (1981). In fact, we published our first cookbook in 1971, **Mothers in the Kitchen**, and have also published **Whole Foods for Babies and Toddlers, Whole Foods for Kids to Cook**, and **Whole Foods from the Whole World**. Like all the mothers before us, we've been trading recipes and sharing ideas for feeding our families for generations. Happily, there are now fathers, partners, and kids in the kitchen, too!

More than two-thirds of the recipes in **Feed Yourself, Feed Your Family** are brand-new, created especially for this book to satisfy your nutritional needs and reflect today's fresh ingredients and cooking trends. One of our core concepts at La Leche League International is: "Good nutrition means eating a well-balanced and varied diet of foods in as close to their natural state as possible." The recipes and foods suggested in these pages reflect that belief.

It's not an accident that we're putting you first in the title. Our goal is to help you stay healthy, with foods that will satisfy you because they taste good and contain the nutrition that your changing body requires. Once you do that, then you can take care of everyone else, from your youngest child to your partner and any other members of your household.

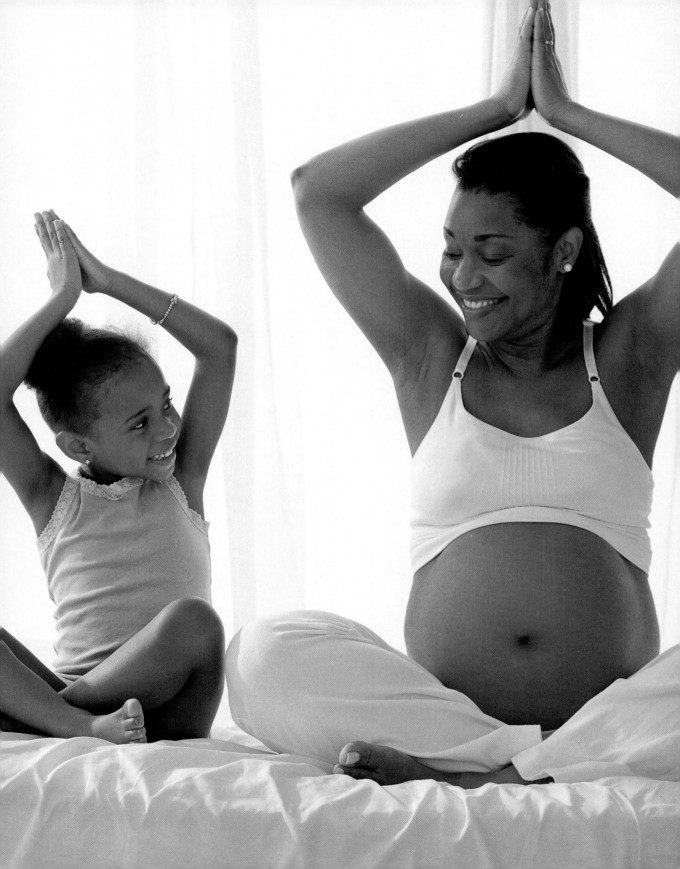

"Salt to Taste": About the Salt in Our Recipes

You'll notice that we've left salt amounts **out** of our original recipes. This isn't an error—we purposely left amounts out because we think it's healthier to salt lightly, as needed, after you taste. Some recipes also contain naturally salty items such as olives or Parmesan cheese. In cases where these savory ingredients are used, you'll find that you can significantly reduce and even eliminate the use of added salt.

Young children (and babies who are starting solids) do not need added salt, and most adults need less than they generally consume. For more information on sodium, see pages 158–62.

About Your Nutritional Needs

There is no magic diet for breastfeeding, nor are there special foods that will cause you to make more milk. However, taking good care of yourself and feeling positive about how and what you eat are key factors in your success. Breastfeeding is different for every mother and child, but one thing is true: if you maintain your health and strength, particularly as you grow accustomed to a breastfeeding lifestyle in the crucial early days, weeks, and months, you're more likely to continue with nursing and give your child all the benefits that come with it, benefits that you will reap as well.

In the chapters that follow, you'll find general information on what key nutrients you should strive to include in your diet, plus food sources and healthy recipes that will help you meet these needs. Our recommendations, thoroughly researched by a registered dietitian who specializes in family nutrition, are mindful of medical and dietary guidelines established by leading organizations such as the American Congress of Obstetricians and Gynecologists (ACOG), the American Academy of Pediatrics (AAP), the American Dietetic Association (ADA), the Centers for Disease Control and Prevention (CDC), the Institute of Medicine of the National Academy of Sciences (IOM), and others.

In later chapters, as your journey through motherhood progresses, we'll include additional information on the nutritional needs and eating habits of your child or children. You'll also find information on solid foods, including the "baby-led" approach that has worked for so many families. (Baby-led is mama-simple, we like to say!)

If you want detailed information on breastfeeding, we recommend you read **The Womanly Art of Breastfeeding**, the classic, bestselling, and always up-to-date comprehensive resource from La Leche League International on making breastfeeding work for you and your baby. You can also visit our website at www.llli.org. Our worldwide community of mothers is waiting to welcome you and your growing family with support and encouragement—and you're bound to find some great recipes, too.

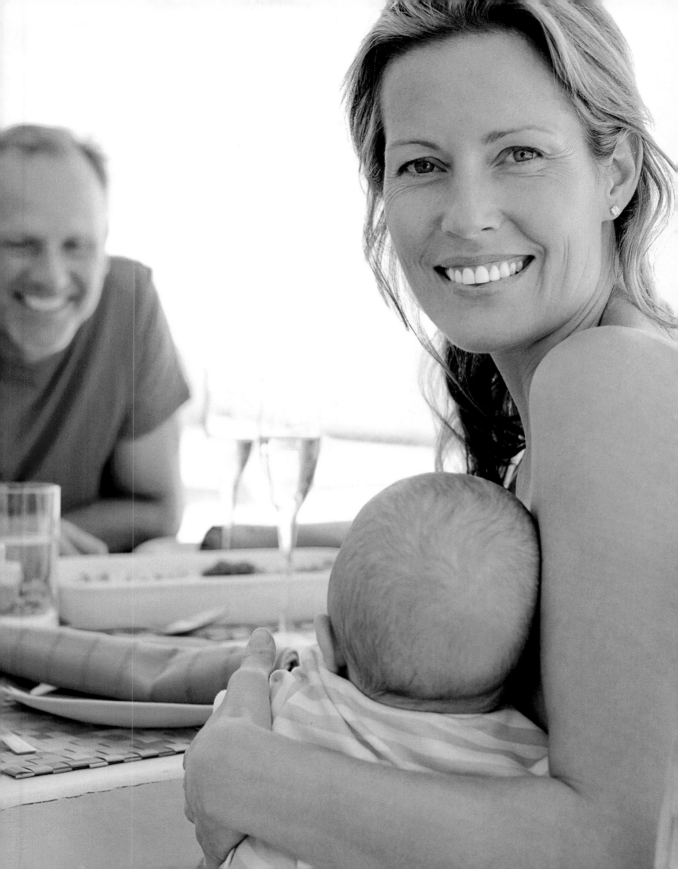

Feed
Yourself,
Feed
Your
Family

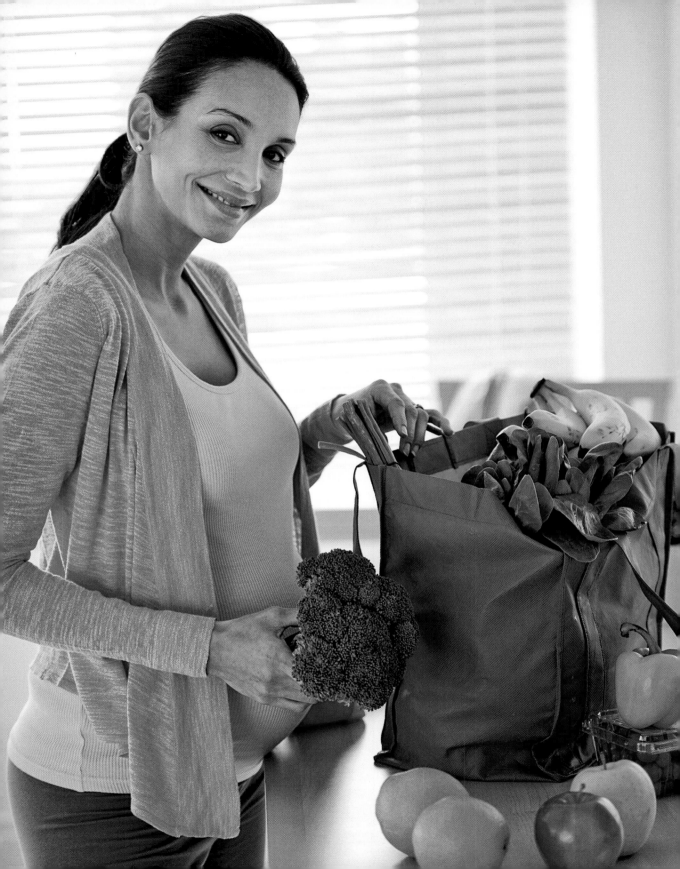

Chapter 1

Getting Ready: Pregnancy, Nutrition, and Breastfeeding

When you are pregnant, you quickly become aware of the connection between what you eat and how it affects your growing baby, and you don't have to work too hard to seek out information. It seems everyone from your doctor to your sister to your sister's best friend has an opinion on what you should have for breakfast, lunch, and dinner.

"Don't drink coffee."

"Our patients do fine with a small amount of coffee—but be careful with fish."

"Stay away from soft cheese. And watch out for the fat content in hard cheese."

"Cheese is packed with calcium you need—why aren't you eating any cheese?"

"Take your prenatal vitamin and you'll be fine."

Eventually you separate the wheat from the chaff (speaking of which, don't forget to eat a lot of whole grains) and grow more confident about your food choices as you strive for a healthy pregnancy. The best advice tends to lie some-where between extreme restriction and complete indulgence. Most experts and research agree, for instance, that a cup of coffee a day is usually okay but limit your caffeine intake to no more than 200 milligrams per day;[1] soft, unpasteurized cheese is among the foods that may contain dangerous listeriosis-causing bacteria and so should be avoided during pregnancy; certain fish, such as swordfish, can carry high levels of mercury and should be off your pregnancy menu; be aware of the high saturated fat and calorie content of hard cheeses such as cheddar; and yes, prenatal vitamins are really important. (We'll return to these and other dos and don'ts later in this chapter.)

If you are reading this book, we're assuming you're already probably taking good care of yourself and your growing baby, and that you're regularly checking in with your physician for advice and information. We're also assuming that since you're planning to breastfeed, you undoubtedly have questions about how what you're eating **now** will impact how you nourish your baby **after** she's born.

As we pointed out in the introduction, there is no magical breastfeeding diet that can be consumed during pregnancy (or afterward) that will guarantee a robust and steady supply of breast milk. However, as you undoubtedly have discovered, maintaining a healthy diet during pregnancy has numerous, excellent benefits for mother and child, whether or not breastfeeding is a goal. And you are more likely to be successful with breastfeeding if you stay healthy and feel strong.

Once you are holding your new nursling in your arms, you'll naturally be less inclined to spend your time planning and preparing meals for yourself and any other members of your household, though your own nutritional needs will still be extremely important! (If you're fast-forwarding to what mealtime will look like after the baby comes, remember that we're here to help. A major goal of this book is to help you balance your dietary needs with those of your nursling, as well as those of other family members.) Therefore, these months and weeks before you give birth and begin breastfeeding are an ideal time to focus more precisely on your diet.

Your Body Is Changing—What About Your Diet?

In the first trimester of a normal pregnancy, a healthy mother-to-be's nutritional and caloric needs won't differ dramatically from what she ate before pregnancy.

If you're eating properly, you'll be able to nourish your growing baby adequately on your prepregnancy diet (with the exception of items to eliminate for safety reasons; see pages 31–32 later in this chapter), though your tastes for certain foods may be altered due to morning sickness or other hormonal changes. It's when you reach the second trimester, however, that the picture begins to change and the increased need for certain macro- and micronutrients, as well as calories, becomes apparent. This phase generally coincides with when you can't button your old jeans!

How much more do you need in terms of nutrients and calories? How much weight should you gain?

Generally, physicians and experts in maternal nutrition recommend that in the second trimester you should up your calories by about 300–350 per day; in your third trimester, you may be advised to increase this by another 100 calories.

As for weight gain, the recommended amount depends on your prepregnancy BMI (body mass index). It simply doesn't make sense to tell a 5'2" woman who is slightly overweight to gain the same amount of weight as a 5'7" woman who is exceedingly thin. Before the widespread use of BMIs, however, pregnant women were frequently given overly general guidelines. Check with your physician to get the number that is right for you, and start with an accurate prepregnancy BMI. (If you are overweight or obese, it's especially important to consult with your physician regarding weight gain.)

While weight gain will vary from woman to woman, less than half of the amount will come from true "baby weight"—that is, the combined weight of the fetus itself, the placenta, and the amniotic fluid. The balance of the weight gain is maternal reproductive tissues such as increased uterus size, blood (its volume increases by 50 percent), breast growth, and additional protein and fat stores. Your heart size alone increases by 12 percent. (We like to think that mothers have the biggest hearts in the world!)

Depending on where you are in your pregnancy, you have undoubtedly noticed that your breasts are changing, beginning with tenderness and soreness that are completely normal. They are also growing rapidly as your body works to make more milk ducts to prepare for breastfeeding. Whether you start out small-breasted or full-figured, the size of your breasts during pregnancy does not impact your ability to nurse your child.

Does your intention to breastfeed mean that you need to supplement or alter those numbers for recommended weight gain and extra calories—in any way? Not at all. Beyond following a healthy and balanced diet during pregnancy, which we will look at in the next section, you don't need to take any special nutritional measures to prepare your body for breastfeeding.

What to Eat Now

You've got your to-do list in hand to get your baby's room or sleeping space ready ahead of time—perhaps it means you'll assemble some furniture, launder some tiny clothing, stockpile diapers, or hang the cow-jumping-over-the-moon picture on the wall. The room, either the nursery or the bedroom where Mom sleeps, will be ready, but what about that other part of your house—the one with the food? Baby's new home can wait a little longer, but let's take a look at what's in your kitchen right now. Whether you're battling morning sickness or you're constantly ravenous (or both), whether you're a reluctant meal planner or absolutely love to cook, **now** is the time to get your food organized.

Naturally, it makes sense to plan around your changing nutritional requirements. In the first trimester, as we pointed out, if you're eating a healthy diet your body doesn't need much more in the way of calories and nutrition. But starting in the second trimester, and as mentioned earlier, your physician will probably recommend about 350 more calories per day until you give birth. (Remember, this calorie recommendation depends on your BMI—check with your doctor to find out how many calories you need to add.) Generally, that translates to a well-planned snack or two, or perhaps a larger portion of a nutritious

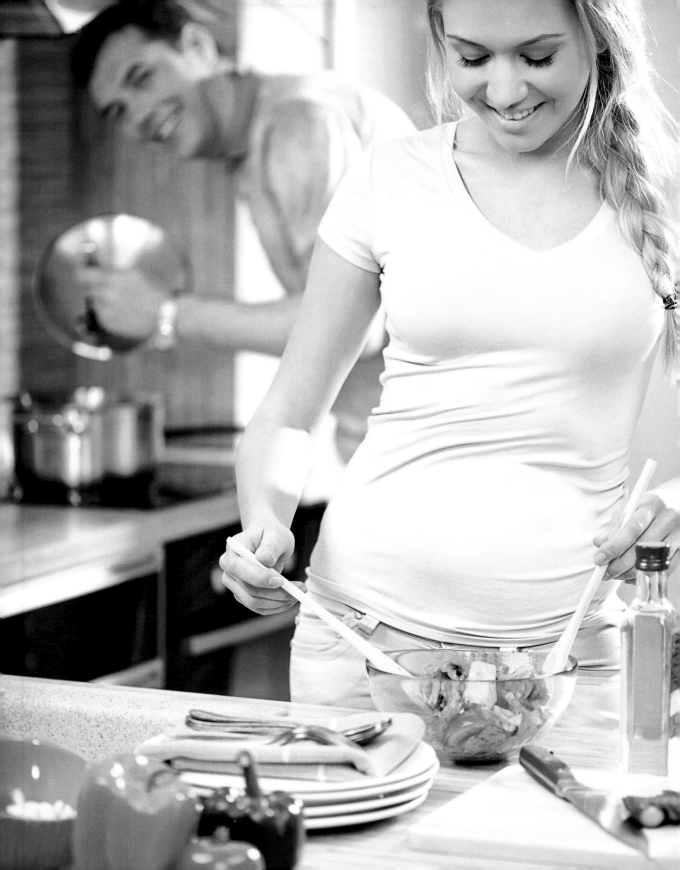

food during mealtime—but not an entire extra meal or double portions of an entrée or dessert. If you overeat, the extra weight gain will not vanish without significant effort. (Yes, you will use extra calories when you are breastfeeding, but postpregnancy weight loss is still harder than pregnancy weight gain. For more on this topic, see page 199.)

A Blueprint for a Lifetime of Healthy Meals

Here's a simple formula for putting together a healthy meal—not just right now but after your baby arrives, and even after your children are old enough to take you out for Mother's Day brunch and when they have kids of their own. This is also a basic but balanced blueprint for assembling just about any family meal. Growing children will require a serving of dairy at each meal, too; if you are pregnant or nursing include three servings of dairy (skim milk is a good choice) for yourself as well. If you or your family does not consume dairy, talk to your doctor or a nutritionist about alternative calcium sources. The chart in the next section includes some nondairy calcium sources, but there are more.

Strive to include each of the following "big three" in every meal you consume.*

1. **Lean protein** (eggs, dairy, meat, fish, legumes)—1 serving.
2. **Vegetables and fruits** (add whole fruit for breakfast)—2 or more servings. (Nutrition experts recommend filling half your plate with veggies and fruit.)
3. **Complex carbohydrates** (from whole-grain bread products or starchy vegetables such as potatoes, corn, and peas)—1 serving. (For more on complex carbohydrates, see the box on pages 14–15.

* For average serving sizes of items such as meat and other protein sources, fruits and vegetables, dairy products, and whole grains, see the sample food listings in the chart on pages 10–11 later in this chapter. When serving sizes are given in weight, it's more helpful to picture an everyday object for a visual cue. Some common examples: 3 ounces of fish, chicken, or beef is about the size of a deck of cards; 1 ounce of hard cheese is about four dice; one serving of fruit is the size of a baseball; $\frac{1}{2}$ cup of veggies is a rounded handful.

Getting the Dietary Components You Need: What, Why, and How Much

Here are some of the major nutrients you should focus on right now, along with some suggested food sources and calorie counts per average serving. Make sure these items are finding their way into your grocery cart and your kitchen. (See our pantry and freezer/refrigerator lists later in this chapter.) Many of these foods can and should also play an important role in your diet after your baby is born. We'll refer you back to this chart in subsequent chapters, with postpartum information on these nutrients.

In some cases, you'll see a comment such as "easiest to get in supplement form." If you are wondering about the food sources versus supplements with regard to calcium and iron, turn to pages 15–17.

A note on adding calories: We don't recommend you get all your extra daily calories from one food source, as it's preferable to vary your diet so your body gets a balance of different nutrients. (And to get 350 calories' worth of vitamin-rich leafy greens, for instance, you'd have to consume about 30 cups of cooked spinach!) Look at the calories per serving of each food on the next pages to mix and match and put together your own balanced 350-calorie boost.*

---

* A note on calories in this chart and elsewhere: These are based on averages used by professional nutritionists, but depending on the cooking techniques, brands, sizes, flavorings, etc. you choose, calorie counts can vary slightly, especially on store-bought items. For instance, a large slice of whole-wheat bread may have more calories than the 69 listed here or a particular brand of low-fat yogurt may have fewer than the 220 we indicate. For an accurate calorie count, check the labels of the products you choose.

	WHAT AND HOW MUCH	WHY IT'S GOOD FOR YOU NOW	WHERE TO FIND IT IN YOUR KITCHEN	CALORIES/KEY NUTRIENTS PER SERVING OF SOME SAMPLE FOODS
PROTEIN	In general, about 70 grams per day; amount depends on the mom's weight and number of babies she is carrying	Gives you building blocks for new tissue synthesis, curbs your hunger, and contains amino acids necessary for fetal growth.	Eggs, poultry, meat, milk, beans, nuts	1 egg: 80 cal, 6 g protein 3 oz chicken (breast): 163 cal, 26 g protein 3 oz beef: 292 cal, 21 g protein 1 cup skim milk: 86 cal, 8 g protein 1 cup soy milk: 79 cal, 6.6 g protein ½ cup cooked chickpeas: 143 cal, 8 g protein ½ cup cooked soybeans: 149 cal, 14 g protein 1 oz almonds: 174 cal, 6 g protein 1 oz peanuts: 164 cal, 7 g protein 1 oz walnuts: 190 cal, 4 g protein 2 tbsp peanut butter: 188 cal, 8 g protein
CALCIUM	1,000 milligrams per day	Bone health (yours and your baby's). Best absorbed from dairy products. Difficult to get daily requirement from vitamin supplement alone—see pages 16–17 on calcium supplements.	Milk, yogurt, cheese (low-fat), fortified cereals, fortified tofu and other fortified soy foods, sardines, salmon, collard greens, beans, peas, seeds, nuts, and whole grains	1 cup skim milk: 86 cal, 300 mg calcium 1 cup low-fat flavored yogurt: 220 cal, 300 mg calcium 1 cup plain yogurt: 127 cal, 452 mg calcium 6 oz Greek yogurt: 225 cal, 150 mg calcium 4 oz soft-serve frozen yogurt: 115 cal, 106 mg calcium 1 cup fortified soy milk: 79 cal, 300 mg calcium 2 sardines: 50 cal, 92 mg calcium Salmon, farmed, 3 oz cooked with dry heat: 151 cal, 10 mg calcium Salmon, wild, 3 oz cooked with dry heat: 119 cal, 38 mg calcium ½ cup chopped boiled fresh collards: 18 cal, 15 mg calcium
IRON	30 milligrams per day	Helps carry oxygen to your baby. While you can get iron from food, it's often easiest to get in supplement form, such as in a prenatal vitamin; see pages 72–73.	Red meat, in particular, but also poultry and pork. Iron-fortified cereals; soybeans, white beans, and lentils; raisins; roasted pumpkin and squash seeds; supplements.*	3.5 oz cooked red meat: 367 cal, 2.13 mg iron 3 oz chicken breast: 163 cal, 0.80–1.00 mg iron ½ cup cooked white beans: 125 cal, 3.30 mg iron ½ cup cooked lentils: 115 cal, 3.25 mg iron ⅓ cup raisins: 150 cal, 1.04 mg iron 1 oz roasted pumpkin seeds: 148 cal, 0.39 mg iron Iron-fortified cereal (for example, ¾ cup Total): 100 cal, 18 mg iron

WHAT AND HOW MUCH	WHY IT'S GOOD FOR YOU NOW	WHERE TO FIND IT IN YOUR KITCHEN	CALORIES/KEY NUTRIENTS PER SERVING OF SOME SAMPLE FOODS	
28 grams per day	Prevents constipation, common during pregnancy. Fiber absorbs water and keeps things moving along regularly in your gastrointestinal tract. Remember to drink water when consuming high-fiber foods.	Fresh fruits and vegetables, whole grains, beans	½ cup cooked beans: 100 cal, 8 g fiber 1 slice whole-wheat bread: 69 cal, 1.9 g fiber 1 cup cooked broccoli: 44 cal, 4.6 g fiber 1 navel orange: 60 cal, 3.1 g fiber ⅓ cup raisins: 150 cal, 2 g fiber	FIBER
600 micrograms per day	Used to develop the baby's neural tube, which becomes its spinal column and brain. Because the neural tube develops in the first month of pregnancy, folate is especially recommended during the first month of pregnancy (and prior to conception), but it is important throughout pregnancy. Occurs naturally in some foods and may be included in a prenatal vitamin.	Chickpeas, lentils, spinach, asparagus, romaine lettuce, orange juice, canned pineapple juice, sunflower seeds, avocado, supplements†	6 oz orange juice: 82 cal, 35 mcg folate 1 cup cooked enriched rice: 170 cal, 130 mcg folate 1 cup cooked spinach: 54 cal, 204 mcg folate ½ cup cooked Great Northern beans: 100 cal, 90 mcg folate	FOLATE

*Note that the amount of calories and iron in a serving of red meat varies based on how lean the cut is. Listed here are averages. Also note that iron in meat is best absorbed when combined with vitamin C. Some examples: a tomato-based meat sauce for pasta; meat garnished with citrus slices or served with cranberry sauce; a glass of orange juice with your meal. Drinking caffeinated beverages with meals will decrease iron absorption.

†Note that only about 50 percent of the natural folate in foods is absorbed and that is why it is necessary in a vitamin supplement as well.

Zinc, Magnesium, and Potassium

Zinc, magnesium, and potassium are also important during pregnancy and breastfeeding. (If you are taking a prenatal supplement, note how much of each it provides.)

Zinc

Zinc assists in DNA and energy production, contributes to a healthy immune system, promotes wound healing, and aids in brain development. During pregnancy, aim for 11 milligrams of zinc. (It goes up slightly, to 12 milligrams, when breastfeeding begins.) Some good sources are meat, fortified breakfast cereals, and the germ or bran of whole grains:

Beef: 3 oz, 9 mg zinc
Lamb: 3 oz, 5 mg zinc
Pork: 3 oz, 4 mg zinc
Fortified breakfast cereal—for example, Total: ½ cup, 34 mg zinc
Wheat germ: 2 tbsp, 2 mg zinc

Though oysters are exceedingly high in zinc (3 ounces provide a whopping 76 milligrams), raw seafood should be avoided during pregnancy (see page 31). Vegetarians need about 50 percent more zinc, as it is not well absorbed from cereals. (For vegetarians, dried seaweed, pumpkin, sesame and sunflower seeds, pine nuts, almonds, and brown rice are also good sources of zinc.)

Magnesium

Magnesium regulates muscle and nerve function, keeps heart rhythm steady, bolsters immunity, and boosts bone development. The recommended amount during pregnancy is 350 milligrams; during nursing, it drops down a bit to 310 milligrams. Do not consume more than 350 milligrams as a supplement, as large doses can cause diarrhea and cramping. (Be aware that some medications, including magnesium hydroxide—sold under various brands as milk of

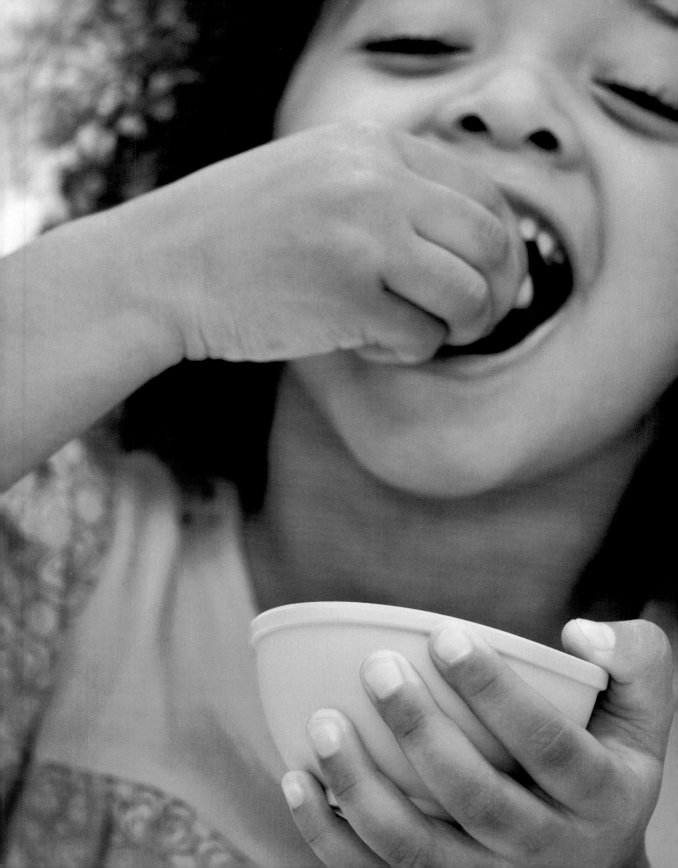

magnesia—used to treat constipation, also contain this mineral.) Some reliable food sources are:

Spinach: 1 cup cooked, 156 mg magnesium
Artichokes: 1 cup, 101 mg magnesium
Brown rice: 1 cup cooked, 84 mg magnesium
Almonds: 1 oz, 78 mg magnesium
Soybeans: ½ cup cooked, 74 mg magnesium
Orange juice: 1 cup, 72 mg magnesium

Potassium

Potassium assists in maintaining a healthy blood pressure. During pregnancy and lactation, the recommended amount is 4,700 milligrams. Fruits and vegetables are the best food sources, though some yogurts can have up to 580 milligrams per 8 ounces (check the label on the brand you buy).

Winter squash: 1 cup, 896 mg potassium
Potato: 1 medium, 610 mg potassium
White beans: ½ cup, 595 mg potassium
Cantaloupe: 1 cup, 473 mg potassium
Orange juice: 1 cup, 496 mg potassium

For additional fruit and vegetable sources of magnesium and potassium not listed above, see page 73.

Carbohydrates: Complex but Not Complicated

All humans need carbohydrates, which provide essential energy. But simple carbohydrates such as table sugar and refined white flour offer little nutritional value and are used up very quickly by the body, without satisfying hunger; this produces a "sugar rush," followed by the low-energy "crash." Simple carbs also crop up in low-nutrient, high-calorie foods such as packaged cookies, soda, candy, and chips. Still, carbohydrates are important. During pregnancy, the fetal brain needs the glucose that is the end product of carbohydrate digestion.

Instead of choosing "empty" carbohydrates with little nutritional value, choose meals and snacks that contain high-fiber **complex** carbohydrates. You'll stay satisfied longer as they release their energy more slowly, and the naturally high fiber content of these foods will help alleviate constipation.

Some sources:

- Whole grains and cereals such as brown rice and oatmeal
- Beans and legumes such as kidney beans, lentils, and split peas
- High-fiber breads and pastas made from whole grains
- Fiber-rich fruits and vegetables such as oranges and broccoli
- Starchy fruits and vegetables such as apples and potatoes
- The recipes in this book ■

Vitamins from Food or Supplements?

It would be so simple if you could get all your essential vitamins during pregnancy from well-balanced meals and snacks. It would be even simpler if you could get everything you needed from a single daily prenatal vitamin supplement that your doctor has recommended. But it's just not possible to rely solely on your diet or a vitamin pill, for reasons we'll explain. The solution, as you'll see, is to both seek out important nutrients in food sources and take the supplement. Let's look at two important vitamins to see why approaching nutrition from two directions is important.

Iron: The Case for Supplements

Iron is vital because your body uses it to make the protein in red blood cells that carries oxygen to your baby. This protein, hemoglobin, is an essential component of your blood. Because your blood volume increases by up to 50 percent during pregnancy (see page 5), you're going to need a lot more iron—30 milligrams daily—to keep your blood supply rich with hemoglobin. (The normal recommended amount is 18 milligrams, which many women don't get.) Where will you get the extra iron?

Three ounces of red meat contain between 3 and 4 milligrams of iron. A cup of edamame (green soybeans) contains about 9 milligrams. Add a slice of whole-wheat bread to our hypothetical plate and you'll consume another 2 to 3 milligrams. (Of course, you can also kick-start your iron consumption by having a bowl of iron-fortified breakfast cereal, which could give you more than 20 milligrams, depending on serving size and brand.) But there's a catch—your body will absorb iron from red meat more effectively than iron from plants, and to optimize your iron absorption, you should consume meat with vitamin C. (This is why in the chart on pages 10–11 we recommended a glass of OJ with your steak.) It's a lot to remember, which is why your prenatal supplement will fill in the gaps.

Some pregnant women find that the iron in a prenatal vitamin contributes to constipation, but this side effect can be lessened. Liquid iron supplements are less constipating because the daily requirement can be divided into 2–3 doses a day. Taking iron supplements with food also tends to reduce constipation, though its absorption may be less effective. (Calcium-containing dairy foods, for instance, can block or reduce iron absorption.)

Taking calcium and iron supplements simultaneously can decrease the absorption of both nutrients. Some women take their calcium in the morning and their iron with dinner with a serving of iron-rich meat or poultry.

Calcium: Drink It and Eat It

Calcium is, of course, a major nutrient that should be consumed during pregnancy for the bone health of mother and baby alike. Pregnant women need at least 1,000 milligrams per day. But unlike iron, it's difficult to get what you need from a supplement, particularly a prenatal supplement, which is attempting to provide so many nutrients in a single pill. Some have no calcium at all, and those that do generally have no more than 200 milligrams. This is because it's difficult to condense large amounts of bulky calcium into pill form to begin with, and a 1,000-milligram dosage in a prenatal supplement would make for an impossibly large pill. (Many women balk at the size of the average prenatal supplement—it's not as big as a bread box, but these are not small pills!)

It's easy, however, to get the additional calcium you need through food sources including milk, cheese, yogurt, and nondairy items such as salmon (our original recipes offer many tasty ways to meet your calcium needs). To get your calcium from dairy products, aim for about three servings per day to help you meet your needs (refer to the chart in this chapter, pages 10–11).

If you are lactose intolerant and do not eat dairy, you may need an additional calcium supplement to reach 1,000 milligrams. Try not to exceed more than 500 milligrams in one dose, as this is about the maximum amount your body can effectively absorb at one time.

Note: Calcium is closely associated with cow's milk because it is a reliable source of this nutrient. However, the consumption of calcium-rich cow's milk and the amount and quality of your breast milk (which also contains calcium) are unrelated. You need extra calcium during pregnancy because your baby's growing bones and teeth require a steady supply of it, but your mature bones and teeth still need calcium, too. If a pregnant woman does not have an extra reserve of calcium, a growing fetus will access the calcium meant to keep the mother's bones and teeth healthy. Weakened bones and tooth decay can result. Additionally, calcium is important for women, as they mature beyond the childbearing years, to reduce the risk of osteoporosis.

DHA: The Brain Builder

Essential fatty acids are fats that cannot be made by the body and therefore must be consumed in your diet. (They are considered essential be-

DHA: The Brain Builder (CONTINUED)

cause without them, your body—and your baby's—cannot function.) In particular, a type of omega-3 polyunsaturated fatty acid known as DHA (short for docosahexaenoic acid) is very important during pregnancy for fetal brain growth and eye development.

About half the fetal brain weight is made up of DHA; at around 24 weeks of gestation, fetal brain growth really takes off and a pregnant mother needs 200–300 milligrams per day of DHA. DHA is found in fish such as salmon (3 ounces contain 740 milligrams), as well as in foods such as DHA-fortified eggs (50 milligrams). However, for pregnant women who don't eat fish, getting enough DHA from food sources can be challenging and supplements can be useful. Check with your health care provider to see if you should be supplementing your diet during pregnancy.

DHA is also essential for brain growth and vision development during a baby's first year of life. Human milk is naturally rich in DHA, and its levels can be increased when a breastfeeding mother consumes more foods containing this important nutrient.

In the Refrigerator and the Pantry: The Hungry Mom's Shopping List

There are many nutritionally dense categories of foods that should stay on your shopping list when you're pregnant, breastfeeding, and beyond. These include:

- **Lean protein:** unprocessed meats, poultry, fish, eggs, legumes
- **Fruits and vegetables:** fresh and frozen (if frozen, with no added syrups or sauces)
- **Low-fat dairy:** reduced-fat or nonfat milk, yogurt, and cheese
- **Whole grains:** fiber-rich breads and cereals, whole-grain crackers or pretzels

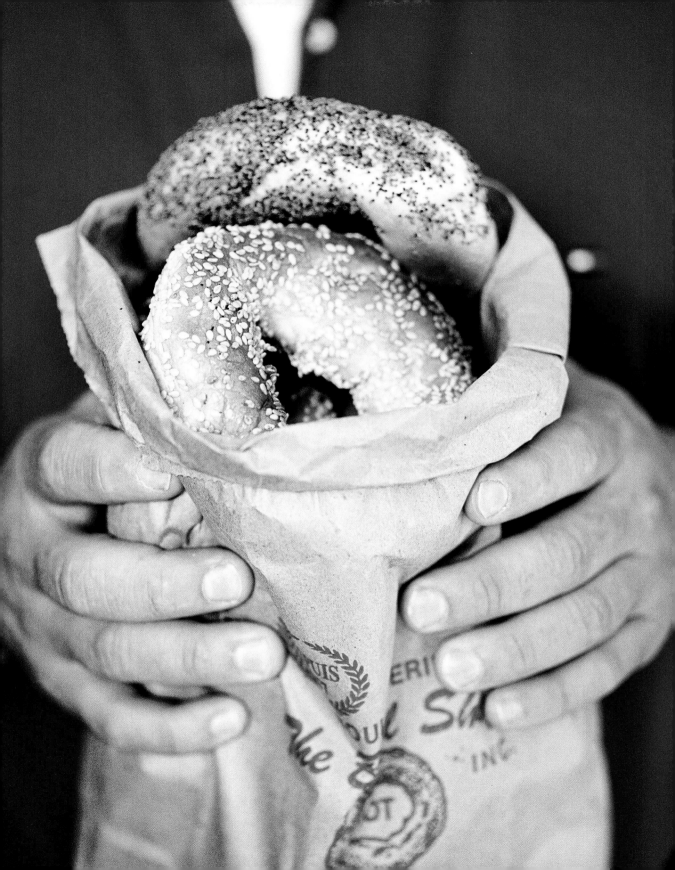

What's in your kitchen right this moment? Maybe you have well-stocked shelves with all the basics and nine varieties of vinegar, or perhaps you aren't much of a planner and you think nothing of running out and buying an onion in mid-sauté.

If you fall into the latter category (and even the best cooks do), you're going to want to rethink those last-minute trips to the market. **Now**—not when you have a newborn who does not care for grocery shopping—is when you should peek in the pantry, the fridge, and the freezer, take stock of your staples (and fresh ingredients), and make sure you have what you'll need to put together a healthy meal without a lot of effort. This list of ingredients and staples is not at all comprehensive, nor will it reflect your personal leanings toward certain types of foods, but if you need some inspiration while making out your grocery list, it's a good start.

IN THE PANTRY

Oils. You may already have **olive oil**, but keep **canola oil**, too. Adults (and children) need a balance of omega-6 and omega-3, two types of essential fatty acids; healthy human cell membranes generally have a 2-to-1 ratio of omega-6 to omega-3. Whether you use it in salad dressings or for cooking or baking, canola oil has the best balance of these two fatty acids, which is why it is often recommended for a rapidly growing fetus, for children, and for breastfeeding mothers.

Dried **herbs, spices**, other **seasonings**. Fresh herbs are terrific, but dried are great for convenience; salt (kosher and sea salts are low in iodine; see page 158).

Vinegars. Balsamic, red, and white.

Flour and other baking ingredients. Whole-wheat (and other whole-grain) and all-purpose flours; a batch of La Leche League Baking Mix (see recipe page 97—this should be stored in the refrigerator or freezer); sugars and other sweeteners; baking soda and baking powder.

Dried **pasta**. Choose whole-wheat and multigrain for complex carbohydrates.

Whole **grains and rice**. Couscous, quinoa, bulgur, barley, oats, cornmeal, wild rice, brown rice, short grain, pearled barley.

Dried **beans and other legumes**. Beans (all are good choices), peas, lentils.

Nuts and seeds. Unsalted—almonds, peanuts, walnuts, pine nuts, sunflower seeds, sesame seeds.

Whole-grain **bread products**. Sandwich bread, tortillas or wraps, pita, crackers, graham crackers, rice cakes, baked pita chips, bread crumbs. To preserve freshness, you may wish to store some bread products in the refrigerator or freeze for later use.

Other **canned and jarred staples**. No- or low-sodium broth, soups, stock; tomatoes (whole, chopped, stewed, pureed, sauce); beans (rinse before using to remove added sodium); tuna (water-packed); peanut butter.

IN THE FREEZER

Frozen **vegetables**.

Frozen **fruit** slices and berries. Tip: Don't toss out that old banana or berries that are about to go over the edge of ripe! Slice the banana into chunks, make sure the berries are washed, and freeze it all. Toss frozen fruit in the blender with yogurt and milk for a quick smoothie later on.

Frozen **pancakes and waffles**. Homemade, that is, not the empty-carb variety you find in the big supermarkets. You can make up a batch of our whole-grain pancakes or waffles and freeze them individually. For a quick breakfast, wrap in foil and heat 8 minutes at 400°F or until done. Defrosted waffles can go in the toaster.

Frozen **pasta**, especially calcium-rich cheese ravioli and tortellini.

Frozen individually wrapped **chicken** breasts, boneless and skinless; lean ground **beef**; ground **turkey**.

Any of our **freezer-friendly recipes**; for a list, see pages 79–80.

Ice cream for a treat—or try **sorbet** or **gelato**!

IN THE REFRIGERATOR

Sauces for pasta (see our recipes for pesto, page 179, and meat sauce, page 227).

Hummus (recipe page 183).

Condiments. Mayonnaise, mustard (Dijon, brown, yellow), horseradish, ketchup, bottled salad dressing (choose low-fat, low-sodium).

Lots of **fruits** and **veggies, salad** fixings, fresh **herbs, lemons,** and **limes.** Not all fruits and vegetables need refrigeration, though it will stop the overripening of that avocado or banana. Remember that items such as apples, onions, potatoes, and squash can have a shelf life of several weeks and are great to have on hand.

Eggs (hard-boil some for quick meals/snacks), **butter,** low-fat **milk** and **yogurt** (plain), hard **cheese, cottage cheese.**

Low-sodium fresh **deli turkey breast slices.**

Olives, chopped jarred **garlic, sun-dried tomatoes.**

Cheese for grating: Parmesan, Pecorino Romano.

Excellent **leftovers** from our recipes!

Read Before You Eat: Nutrition Labels

You're on the go, and you're starving (and thirsty), as you often seem to be during your pregnancy, so you pop into a mini-mart and look for something healthful. A huge selection of energy bars—perfect, you think. You devour one and then look at the label. You just ate 240 calories, more than half of which were from fat, and there was more sugar involved than fiber or protein. You washed it down with what you thought was a healthful beverage—a vitamin-enriched drink that has 80 calories per serving—but that one bottle you just chugged actually contained three servings. In this case, you would have been better off with a nut-packed candy bar and a plain bottle of water.

Read the labels. Now more than ever, train yourself to look at the nutritional labels on the boxes, bags, and cans of everything that you consume. If there is an ingredient or an amount that is stumping you, find out what it means; it's going into your body, and your baby is eating it, too. In addition to ingredients, pay attention to serving size. Most of us know that food companies give the information for a single serving on their packaging, but many items are not packaged as single servings. Visit www.fda.gov/food/labelingnutrition/consumerinformation/ucm078889 .htm for a primer on label reading.

Of course, when you're so hungry you could eat the entire rack of snacks at the cash register, you may not be focused on the fine print. Avoid hunger that drives you into the mini-mart in the first place by eating well and carrying your own healthy snacks. See the section "Snacks That Make Sense," following, for some suggestions. ■

Snacks That Make Sense

If you're working during the day or busy at home with another child or two, you want no-cook snacks that will satisfy your hunger. If a snack food leaves you hungry for more, rethink your choice—it's probably not as nutritionally dense as other options. You'll do best when you combine nutrients such as proteins and carbohydrates. Together, they'll release more slowly into your bloodstream and will take the edge off your hunger until your next meal.

Here are some of our favorite snack ideas that will go where you go and involve no cooking, just smart shopping. Stash these items (the ones that don't require refrigeration) in your desk, your pocketbook, or your car, and keep fresh ingredients in your home kitchen or the office fridge. And don't forget a refillable water bottle. (For information on hydration during pregnancy, see "Quenching Your Thirst," later in this chapter.)

- An apple and a small handful of almonds
- Peanut butter or almond butter on a slice of whole-grain toast
- Greek-style low- or nonfat yogurt (higher in protein than most other yogurts) and fresh berries

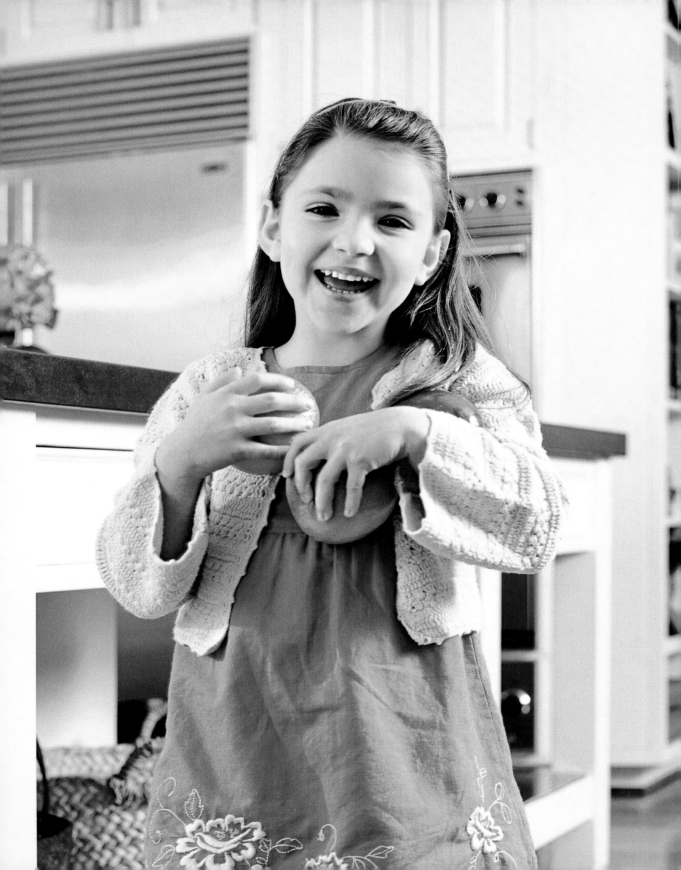

- Whole-grain pretzels or crackers and nuts
- Mini rice cakes (try brown rice) with hummus or nut butter
- Roasted chickpeas
- Hulled, unsalted sunflower seeds
- A bowl of cereal and skim milk (it's not just for breakfast)
- Homemade trail mix mixed from low-fat granola cereal, raisins, nuts, and dried fruit
- Skim milk and a banana
- Deli turkey slices, whole-grain crackers, and baby carrots
- A hard-boiled egg
- Some Hummus (see recipe page 183) and a few whole-grain crackers

The 15/5 Snack Rule

Trying to determine if what you're about to munch on is a good choice? Developed by a nutrition professional, these four steps help you balance carbohydrates and fats.[2]

1. Look at the food label.
2. Determine the serving size.
3. Look at the total carbohydrate on the food label. An appropriate snack will have around 15 grams or less per serving.
4. Look at the total fat on the food label. An appropriate snack will have 5 grams or less. For example:

Rice Cakes—Chocolate Crunch Flavored

SERVING SIZE: 1 rice cake (15 grams)
TOTAL CARBOHYDRATE: 11 grams
TOTAL FAT: 1 gram

Meals That Give You More

At the end of this chapter, you'll find tempting recipes for meals such as Roasted Shrimp with Grape Tomatoes and Summer Squash, Tabbouleh (Bulgur and Lentil Salad), and even a sweet treat and La Leche League International favorite, an old-fashioned Banbury Tart. There are hearty breakfast foods, including our Pepper and Spinach Frittata, and main courses that work as lunch or dinner, such as Grilled Chicken Chopped Salad. (The frittata makes a great lunch or dinner, too!)

But of course, you don't need a recipe for every meal. Here are some basic ideas involving minimal cooking, with maximum nutrition, for breakfast, lunch, and dinner. Use your imagination and keep in mind our blueprint for a healthy meal (see page 8) as you add sides and beverages to round out your choices.

BREAKFAST IDEAS

- Oatmeal (regular or quick-cooking), with fresh fruit and nonfat or low-fat yogurt
- Eggs, whole-grain toast, and calcium-fortified orange juice
- Whole-grain waffles or pancakes with fruit (make your own and freeze—see page 154)
- Whole-grain cereal, skim milk, and fruit
- Whole-grain muffin, yogurt, and berries (see our freezer-friendly muffin recipes on pages 98 and 146)

LUNCH IDEAS

- Turkey breast slices, low-fat cheese, and grated carrots in a whole-grain pita or wrap
- Cottage cheese, shredded carrots, chopped cucumbers, and sunflower seeds in a whole-grain wrap

- Low-sodium barley and vegetable soup, whole-grain crackers, and green salad
- Whole-grain pasta with chopped chicken breast and veggies

DINNER IDEAS

- Salmon with vegetables and brown rice
- Whole-grain spaghetti and turkey meatballs in tomato sauce
- Soup made with chicken, beans, and vegetables
- Stir-fried beef and broccoli
- Cheese tortellini and tomato sauce

If You Don't Eat Meat

Though many of the meal suggestions above feature meat, fish, and poultry, we recognize that many pregnant women who plan to breastfeed are committed vegetarians or vegans, and their partners and families may be as well.

You'll find a number of meatless main dish recipes in these pages, such as Slow Cooker Vegetarian Chili (page 136), Quinoa Pilaf with White Beans, Feta Cheese, and Summer Vegetables (page 139), Tortilla Pie with Black Beans and Cheddar (page 48), and many more (see list below), plus dozens of hearty vegetable side dishes, such as Roasted Root Vegetables (page 52), in addition to recipes that can be adapted and made without meat.

If this is your first pregnancy as a vegetarian or vegan, consult with your health care provider or a nutrition professional to make sure you're getting the additional iron, zinc, and vitamin B_{12} that you need during this stage and after your baby is born.

Vegetarian Main Dish Recipes

Quenching Your Thirst

Consuming enough fluids (and the right ones) during pregnancy is part of a healthy prenatal diet. Water is vital because your body is processing it rapidly to accommodate fetal growth and increased blood volume. It will also help you avoid constipation, a common symptom during pregnancy. Check with your health care provider to find out how much water you should be drinking (the one-size-fits-all rule of eight glasses a day doesn't necessarily apply). Other drinks such as juices, milk, coffee, tea, and carbonated beverages all count toward your daily fluid intake. In addition, most fruits and vegetables have naturally high water content and can help you stay hydrated (though you should still drink water).

The need to urinate increases as pregnancy progresses—the growing uterus puts pressure on your bladder, and the kidneys work overtime to accommodate

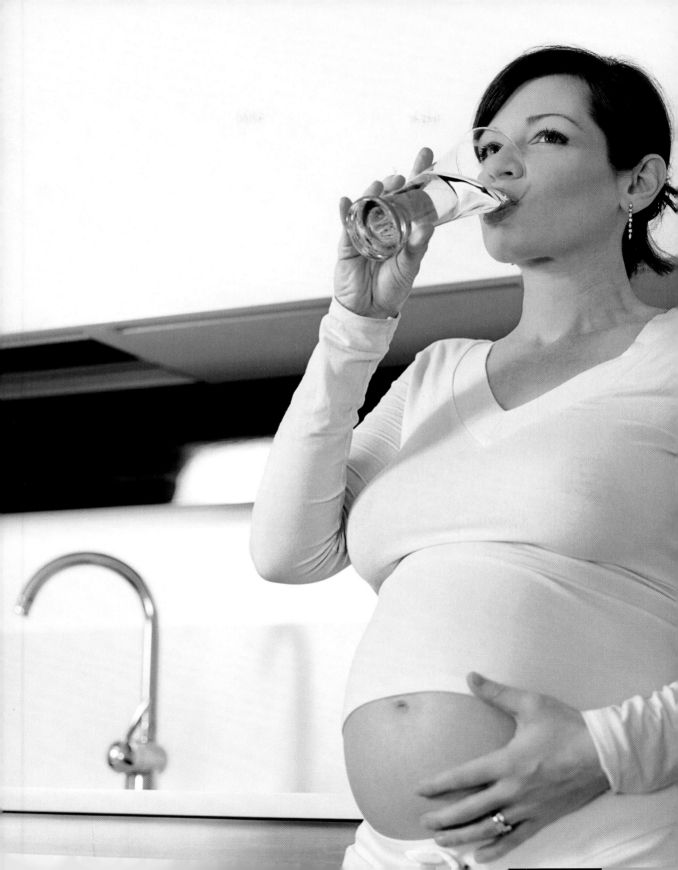

your body's increased blood volume. It's tempting to avoid drinking water, but it's better to make an extra pit stop or two than to risk dehydration. (Remember that this phase—like so many in pregnancy and motherhood—is temporary.) Your urine should be pale; if it's dark yellow in color, then you're not getting enough to drink.

If you have not done so, talk to your health care provider about caffeine intake. As noted earlier, there is scant evidence to suggest that moderate caffeine consumption will lead to miscarriage or other serious complications, but some pregnant women choose to remove caffeine from their diets entirely. (To reiterate, "moderate" is defined as 200 milligrams per day, the amount in about two 8-ounce cups of coffee, but check the caffeine content of your preferred brand, as it can vary. For information on caffeine consumption during breastfeeding, see **The Womanly Art of Breastfeeding**, as well as page 76 of this book.)

If you love certain popular coffee drinks, be aware that sometimes these rich, sugary, whipped-cream-topped beverages have more in common with full-fat milk shakes than with coffee. Though you can order a caffeine-free version, consider the calories; it would be fairly easy to consume **more** than your extra 350 calories by sipping just one of these fancy coffee drinks a day!

Brewed tea generally has less caffeine than coffee, but check the content so you know precisely what you are consuming. Not every caffeine-free herbal tea and drink should be considered totally safe during pregnancy, despite claims of "natural," unprocessed ingredients. Some herbs in large quantities, for instance, have been shown to stimulate the uterus, including some forms of chamomile. Citrus peel, ginger, lemon balm, and rose hip are considered safe; check with your doctor for more information. Herbal teas, like herbal remedies, are not regulated by the FDA. (For some additional information on herbs and breastfeeding, see page 125.)

The negative effects of alcohol on fetal development are well documented; check with your health care provider for more information. Leading obstetric and pediatric organizations remain unanimously firm in their long-held positions: no amount of alcohol consumption during pregnancy should be considered safe. (For information on alcoholic beverages and breastfeeding, see **The Womanly Art of Breastfeeding**, and pages 76–77 of this book.)

Should You Eat That When You're Pregnant?

There are certain foods that have been linked to serious illness or complications during pregnancy, primarily because they carry bacteria that can cause illnesses such as salmonella and listeriosis. (Other infections, such as toxoplasmosis, can be caused by bacteria found in cat waste, which is why pregnant women are always cautioned against changing a pet's litter box; pets such as birds and turtles can also pass along salmonella.) These illnesses can affect anyone, but they are particularly dangerous for pregnant women, as the bacteria can be transmitted to a fetus and impair development or cause miscarriage or stillbirth.

Salmonella

The bacteria that cause salmonella live in human and animal intestines and are spread through feces. During the butchering process, salmonella can infect meat and poultry, though thorough cooking will kill the bacteria. **Avoid raw meats, raw poultry, raw (unpasteurized) milk, raw fish (sushi), raw eggs, unwashed fruits and vegetables, and contaminated water. Practice safe handling of raw and cooked foods, including cooking food to correct temperatures and observing proper storage; wash hands thoroughly.**

Listeriosis

This food-borne illness can be especially serious for pregnant women and newborns. Listeria, which also occurs in soil, plants, water, and animals, can be found in these foods, which should be avoided: **soft, unpasteurized cheeses (Brie, Camembert, blue-veined cheeses, feta, queso fresco, queso blanco, queso panela);* any products made with raw, unpasteurized milk; packaged hot dogs, packaged deli meats, and meat or fish pâtés—these types of**

---

* A few recipes in this book call for feta or goat cheese. Please note that we specify **pasteurized** varieties only—read labels carefully to confirm pasteurization. Pasteurized (usually domestic) goat and feta cheeses are available in most large supermarkets.

products can become contaminated after they are processed and before they reach the consumer.

Your health care provider can give you a more comprehensive listing of foods to avoid while pregnant. If you have food allergies or sensitivities (see pages 126–28) or other conditions requiring you to follow a certain diet, you undoubtedly have your own list of foods that are on your "don't eat" list.

A Fishy Dilemma Resolved

Though fish can be an excellent source of omega-3 fatty acids (see "DHA: The Brain Builder" on pages 17–18), we've just cautioned you against sushi, since raw or undercooked fish can make you and your baby sick. And now we're about to tell you a little more about several varieties of fish to avoid when pregnant because they can contain high levels of mercury.

Methylmercury is an environmental contaminant that gets into our water supply; small fish eat mercury-contaminated plants and insects, and larger fish feed on the small ones. Fish such as swordfish, king mackerel, shark, and tilefish have the highest levels of mercury, which can be very harmful to fetal development, and should be avoided.

Still, fish is an excellent source of DHA (and because of its bony nature, fish can be high in calcium; the canning process softens the bones to the point of near invisibility and makes them digestible). Here's a short list of safe fish.

- Salmon
- Shrimp
- Sardines
- Pollack
- Catfish
- Tilapia
- Canned light tuna (12 ounces per week)
- Albacore tuna (6 ounces per week)

For more information on safe fish consumption during breastfeeding, see page 125–26.

You'll find the following fish and seafood recipes in this book:

- Baked Salmon with Apricot Glaze, page 178
- Roasted Salmon with Light Horseradish Sour Cream Sauce, page 35
- Soy-Lime Marinated Salmon, page 133
- Roasted Shrimp with Grape Tomatoes and Summer Squash, page 36
- Shrimp Scampi Whole-Grain Pasta Toss, page 135
- Whole-Wheat Spaghetti with Anchovies and Cauliflower, page 90
- Mounds of Mussels, page 92
- Crab Tostadas, page 91
- Fish Chowder, page 229

Not Bad for the Reasons Above, but Not So Good, Either

There are plenty of widely available foods that are considered safe to eat, as they don't harbor threatening bacteria, cause food-borne illness, or exacerbate food allergies or sensitivities. But over the long term, some of these "safe" foods may not be so safe after all, because they consist of nutrient-poor calories.

Many mothers will claim, "I ate my healthiest diet when I was pregnant." Get into the habit of eating well now and reaping the benefits, and it will be easier to follow a healthy diet later and share your good habits. Avoid letting these common culprits creep onto your plate with regularity (read labels), and they'll stay out of your family's diet, too.

- **High-fat foods.** Foods rich in saturated fat include burgers, pizza, burritos, and other fast food; fatty meats such as bacon; and full-fat dairy foods such as cheese and ice cream. Some foods that may not appear to be high in fat may contain trans fats, which raise cholesterol (read ingredient labels—hydrogenated or partially hydrogenated oils signal trans fat).*

- **High-sugar foods and "empty" carbohydrates.** These may include baked goods made with refined white flour (packaged cookies, donuts, white bread, bagels), sugary sodas and beverages (including "juice beverages," which are not 100 percent juice, and excessive amounts of fruit juice), candy, chips, and sugary breakfast cereal.
- **High-sodium foods.** Some examples include fast food and restaurant foods, prepackaged convenience foods, and snack foods such as pretzels and crackers (see pages 158–62 for more on sodium).

As you can see, because high fat, sugar, and sodium content is often characteristic of fast food, prepackaged foods, convenience foods, and highly processed foods, the best way to avoid them entirely is to make your own food, eat in establishments where healthy and natural foods are the focus of the menu, and be prepared with your own stash of pantry staples, nutritious snacks, and high-quality leftovers.

If you fall in love with one of our recipes, double it and store the extras, or make sure that you always have the staple ingredients on hand. Stockpile your refrigerator, freezer, and cupboards with good food. You'll be feeding your new baby soon enough. Take the time now to make sure you're well fed, too!

* Though the label may say zero grams of trans fat, manufacturers do not need to disclose trans fat content if the amount is less than 0.5 grams per serving, and you may be unaware that you've consumed it. For example, if you eat three or four servings of most microwave popcorn made with partially hydrogenated oils, you have probably just eaten about 2 grams of trans fat.

Roasted Salmon with Light Horseradish Sour Cream Sauce

SERVES 4

2 fennel bulbs, cored and thinly sliced

1 red onion, thinly sliced

1 tablespoon extra-virgin olive oil

Salt and freshly ground black pepper

4 6-ounce skinless salmon fillets

½ cup reduced-fat sour cream

1 tablespoon prepared horseradish

1 teaspoon Dijon mustard

1. Preheat the oven to 450°F.

2. In a large rimmed baking sheet, toss the fennel and onion with the oil and a pinch each of salt and pepper until evenly coated. Spread in a single layer. Roast for 15 minutes, then push the vegetables to one side of the pan.

3. Sprinkle salt and pepper over the salmon and arrange in a single layer on the other side of the pan. Roast until the fish is just opaque throughout and the vegetables are just tender, about 10 minutes longer.

4. Meanwhile, stir together the sour cream, horseradish, and mustard in a small bowl.

5. Spoon the horseradish sauce over the salmon and serve with the vegetables.

Roasted Shrimp with Grape Tomatoes and Summer Squash

SERVES 4

1 lemon

3 tablespoons extra-virgin olive oil

1 garlic clove, finely chopped

¼ teaspoon dried oregano

1 pint grape tomatoes

2 large summer squash, trimmed and cut into ½-inch-thick rounds

Salt and freshly ground black pepper

1 pound large shrimp (16 to 20 count), shelled and deveined

¼ cup Kalamata olives, pitted and chopped

6 ounces baby spinach

1. Preheat the oven to 450°F.

2. Zest the lemon directly over a large bowl. Cut the lemon into wedges and reserve. To the zest, add the oil, garlic, and oregano. Pour half of the mixture onto a rimmed baking sheet.

3. Add the tomatoes and squash to the baking sheet and toss to coat. Sprinkle salt and pepper all over and roast until the tomatoes begin to collapse and the squash begins to brown, about 15 minutes.

4. Meanwhile, add the shrimp and olives to the bowl with the remaining oil mixture and season with pepper. Toss to coat. Add to the pan with the vegetables, spreading everything in an even layer. Roast 5 minutes or until the shrimp are cooked through.

5. Divide the spinach among serving plates and spoon over it the shrimp mixture with all of its juices. Serve with lemon wedges.

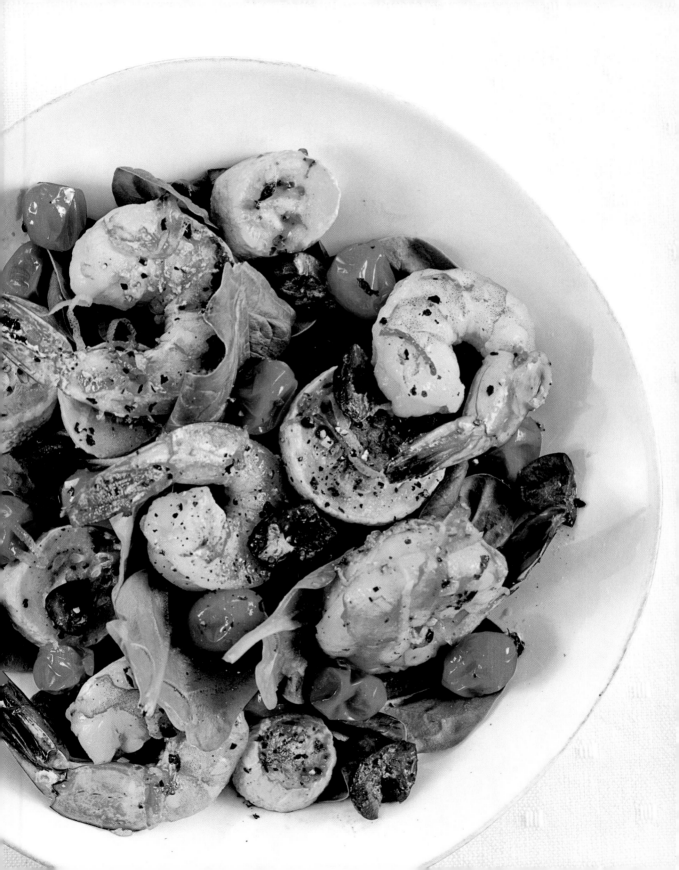

Chicken, Carrot, and Potato Mild Curry

SERVES 4

4 carrots, cut into ½-inch chunks

4 Yukon gold potatoes, scrubbed and cut into ½-inch chunks

2 tablespoons canola oil

1 large onion, finely chopped

3 garlic cloves, finely chopped

1 1-inch piece fresh ginger, peeled and finely chopped

Salt and freshly ground black pepper

1 pound boneless, skinless chicken breasts, cut into ½-inch chunks

2 teaspoons ground cumin

1 teaspoon ground turmeric

1 13.5-ounce can light coconut milk

1. Combine the carrots, potatoes, and ¼ cup water in a medium microwave-safe bowl. Cover with plastic wrap, poke a few holes in the plastic, and microwave on high for 8 minutes or until tender enough for a knife to pierce through easily.

2. Meanwhile, heat the oil in a large, wide saucepan over medium-high heat. Add the onion and cook, stirring occasionally, until golden brown, about 5 minutes. Stir in the garlic and ginger and cook, stirring, for 1 minute.

3. Sprinkle salt and pepper all over the chicken and add to the pan. Cook, stirring occasionally, until no longer pink on the outside, about 4 minutes. Add the cumin and turmeric and cook, stirring, for 1 minute.

4. Add the coconut milk and the carrot mixture with its liquid. Bring to a boil, then reduce the heat to medium and simmer, stirring occasionally, until the chicken is cooked through, about 10 minutes. Season to taste with salt and pepper.

Favorite Chicken Noodle Soup

SERVES 12

4 quarts canned lower-sodium chicken broth

1 whole (3½-pound) chicken, cut into 8 pieces

1 medium onion, chopped

4 carrots, thinly sliced

4 celery stalks, sliced

2 tablespoons (¼ stick) butter

2 cups sliced mushrooms

1 garlic clove, minced

1 tablespoon fresh lemon juice

8 ounces dried wide egg noodles

¼ cup finely chopped fresh flat-leaf parsley leaves

1. Combine the chicken broth and chicken in a heavy large pot. Bring to a boil over high heat, then reduce the heat to medium. Cover partially and simmer, skimming any foam that rises to the surface, until the chicken is cooked through, about 20 minutes. Use tongs to transfer the chicken to a large bowl. Skim any fat from the chicken broth.

2. Add the onion, carrots, and celery to the broth. Bring to a boil, then reduce the heat to maintain a steady simmer. Cook until the vegetables are tender, about 10 minutes.

3. When the chicken is cool enough to handle, discard the skin and bones. Shred the meat into bite-size pieces.

4. Melt the butter in a large skillet over medium-high heat. Add the mushrooms and garlic and cook, stirring occasionally, until browned, about 5 minutes. Remove from the heat and stir in the lemon juice.

5. Add the noodles, parsley, chicken, and mushrooms to the simmering broth. Cook, stirring occasionally, until the noodles are tender, about 5 minutes. Season to taste with salt and pepper.

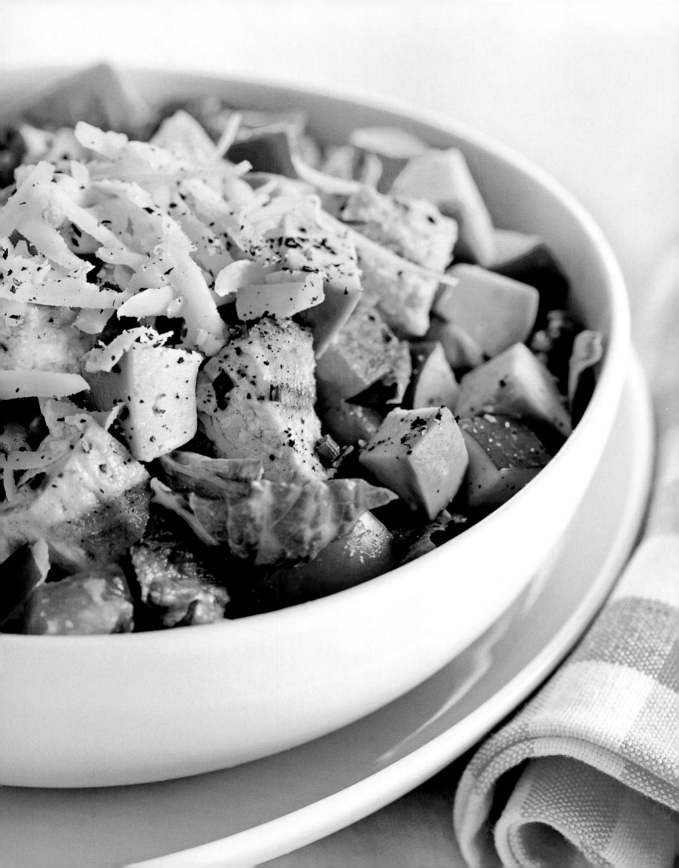

Grilled Chicken Chopped Salad

SERVES 4

2 tablespoons extra-virgin olive oil

1 garlic clove, finely chopped

1 tablespoon chopped fresh rosemary leaves

1 pound chicken cutlets

Salt and freshly ground black pepper

½ cup buttermilk

2 tablespoons mayonnaise

1 tablespoon fresh lemon juice

1 tablespoon Dijon mustard

2 tablespoons snipped chives

2 romaine lettuce hearts, chopped

2 tomatoes, cored, seeded, and diced

1 Gala or Fuji apple, cored and diced

1 avocado, halved, pitted, peeled, and diced

¼ cup grated sharp cheddar cheese

1. Combine the oil, garlic, and rosemary in a large resealable plastic bag. Add the chicken and turn to coat. Refrigerate until ready to cook, up to 8 hours.

2. Heat an outdoor grill or preheat a grill pan to medium high.

3. Transfer the chicken to the hot grill and season with salt and pepper. Grill, flipping once, until cooked through, about 8 minutes. Transfer to a cutting board and let stand for 5 minutes. Cut into slices or bite-size chunks.

4. Whisk together the buttermilk, mayonnaise, lemon juice, mustard, chives, and a generous pinch each of salt and pepper in a large bowl.

5. Add the lettuce, tomato, and apple to the buttermilk mixture and toss until evenly coated. Divide among serving plates. Top with the avocado, cheese, and chicken.

Turkey Shepherd's Pie with Sweet Potatoes

SERVES 12

3 medium sweet potatoes

2 tablespoons canola oil

1 pound ground turkey

Salt and freshly ground black pepper

2 tablespoons all-purpose flour

1 cup lower-sodium chicken broth

1 pound parsnips, peeled and chopped

3 celery stalks, finely chopped

1 medium onion, finely chopped

2 cups frozen peas

¼ cup reduced-fat (2%) milk, warmed

1 tablespoon butter

1. Pierce the sweet potatoes all over with a fork. Place on a microwave-safe dish and microwave on high for 7 minutes. Turn the potatoes over and microwave until very tender, about 8 minutes longer.

2. Meanwhile, heat 1 tablespoon oil in a large skillet over medium-high heat. Add the turkey and sprinkle with salt and pepper. Cook, stirring occasionally and breaking the meat into small chunks, until no longer pink, about 5 minutes.

3. Stir the flour into the turkey and cook, stirring, for 1 minute. Stir in the broth and bring to a boil. Cook, stirring, until the mixture thickens slightly, about 2 minutes. Transfer the turkey to a 3-quart baking dish and spread in an even layer.

4. Preheat the oven to 425°F.

5. Heat the remaining oil in the same skillet over medium heat. Stir in the parsnips, celery, onion, and ¼ cup water. Cover and cook, stirring occasionally, until the vegetables are browned and tender, about 15 minutes. Stir in the frozen peas and season to taste with salt and pepper. Pour the vegetable mixture over the turkey mixture and spread in an even layer.

6. When the sweet potatoes are cool enough to handle, cut them in half. Use a spoon to scoop out the flesh from the skins; discard the skins.

Turkey Shepherd's Pie with Sweet Potatoes

Transfer the sweet potatoes to a large bowl and mash coarsely with a potato masher or fork. Stir in the milk and butter and season to taste with salt and pepper. Continue mashing until well blended. Spread the potatoes evenly over the vegetables.

7. Bake, uncovered, until the top is lightly browned, about 20 minutes.

Old-Fashioned Kerwin* Chili

SERVES 8

2 pounds lean ground beef

Salt and freshly ground black pepper

1 garlic clove

1 medium onion, finely chopped

2 15-ounce cans kidney beans, rinsed and drained

1 28-ounce can whole tomatoes in juice

1 6-ounce can tomato paste

2 tablespoons no-salt-added chili powder

⅛ teaspoon cayenne pepper, optional

½ teaspoon Worcestershire sauce

*Mary Ann Kerwin is a co-founder of LLLI.

1. Heat a large, heavy saucepan over high heat. Add the beef, season with salt and pepper, and cook, stirring occasionally and breaking the meat into small chunks, until browned, about 8 minutes.

2. Add in the garlic and cook, stirring, until golden, about 1 minute. Stir in the onion, beans, tomatoes, tomato paste, chili powder, cayenne, and Worcestershire sauce. Bring to a boil, stirring occasionally and breaking up the whole tomatoes, then reduce the heat to medium low.

3. Simmer, stirring occasionally, until the flavors meld, at least 15 minutes and up to 30 minutes. For a thinner consistency, stir in water.

Bacon and Spinach Pasta

SERVES 10

8 slices bacon

1½ pounds linguine

9 tablespoons extra-virgin olive oil

8 ounces mushrooms, quartered

4 garlic cloves, thinly sliced

Salt and freshly ground black pepper

12 ounces baby spinach*

2 teaspoons chopped fresh oregano leaves

2 tablespoons chopped fresh basil leaves

2 cups freshly grated Pecorino Romano or Parmesan cheese

*Even if you purchase prewashed spinach, if you are pregnant food safety advocates recommend that you wash and dry packaged spinach thoroughly.

1. Bring a large pot of water to a boil.

2. Cook the bacon according to the package directions. When cool, crumble.

3. Cook the pasta according to the package directions and drain.

4. Meanwhile, heat 3 tablespoons oil in a large skillet over medium-high heat. Add the mushrooms and garlic and a pinch each of salt and pepper. Cook, stirring occasionally, until the mushrooms are tender and the garlic golden, about 6 minutes. Gently stir in the spinach and cook until wilted, about 2 minutes. Stir in the oregano, basil, remaining 6 tablespoons oil, and another pinch each of salt and pepper.

5. Divide the pasta among serving plates. Top with the mushroom mixture, then with the bacon and cheese.

Pepper and Spinach Frittata

SERVES 4

7 large eggs

Salt and freshly ground black pepper

2 tablespoons extra-virgin olive oil

1 small onion, diced

1 red bell pepper, stemmed, seeded, and diced

1 orange bell pepper, stemmed, seeded, and diced

1 yellow bell pepper, stemmed, seeded, and diced

6 ounces baby spinach

1 cup grated Pecorino Romano cheese

1. Arrange an oven rack 6 inches from the broiler heat source. Preheat the broiler.

2. Beat the eggs with a pinch of salt and pepper in a large bowl until blended.

3. Heat 1 tablespoon oil in a 12-inch ovenproof nonstick skillet over medium heat. Add the onion and cook, stirring occasionally, until just softened, about 4 minutes. Add the red, orange, and yellow bell peppers. Season with salt and pepper and cook, stirring occasionally, until lightly browned and softened, about 8 minutes. Add the spinach, season with salt and pepper, and cook, stirring, until just wilted. Scrape the mixture into the eggs.

4. Wipe out the skillet with a paper towel and heat the remaining oil in it over medium heat. Add the egg mixture. When the eggs set on the bottom and around the sides, gently lift with a spatula to let the uncooked egg run under. Repeat until the eggs are almost set.

5. Sprinkle the cheese over the top and transfer to the broiler. Broil until the eggs are completely set and the top is golden brown, about 5 minutes.

6. Let cool in the pan for 5 minutes. Loosen the edges with a spatula and slide out of the pan onto a serving plate. Cut into wedges.

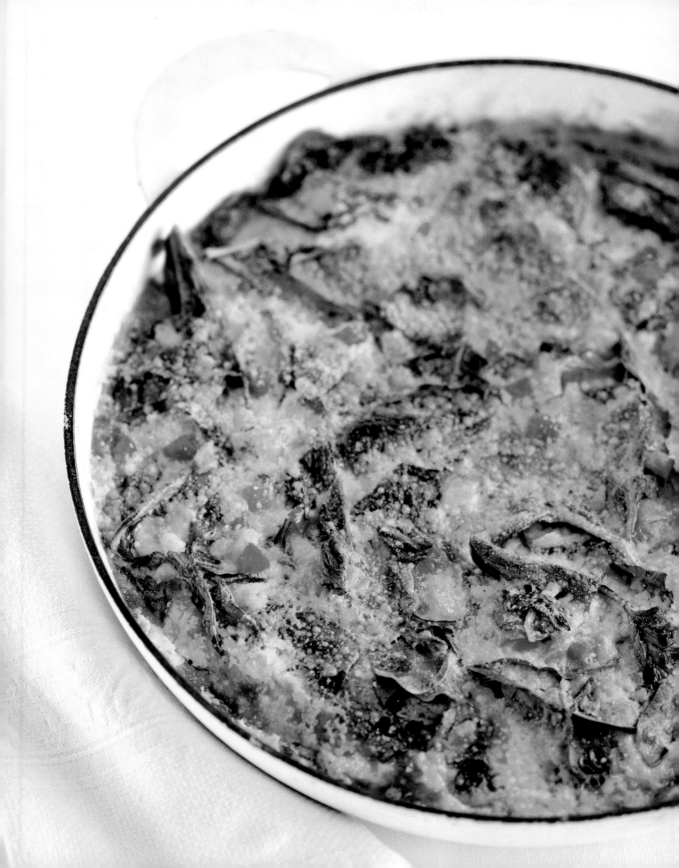

Tortilla Pie with Black Beans and Cheddar

SERVES 4

2 tablespoons canola oil

1 medium onion, finely chopped

1 yellow bell pepper, stemmed, seeded, and finely chopped

2 garlic cloves, finely chopped

3 large tomatoes, cored, seeded, and chopped

1 tablespoon tomato paste

Salt and freshly ground black pepper

9 corn tortillas

¾ cup reduced-fat sour cream

1 cup shredded sharp cheddar cheese

¼ cup packed fresh cilantro leaves, chopped

1 15-ounce can black beans, rinsed and drained

1 cup fresh corn kernels

1. Preheat the oven to 400°F.

2. Heat the oil in a large, deep ovenproof skillet over medium-high heat. Add the onion and pepper and cook, stirring occasionally, until browned and just tender, about 6 minutes. Add the garlic and cook, stirring, for 1 minute. Add the tomatoes and tomato paste, season with salt and pepper, and cook, stirring occasionally, until the mixture is thickened but the tomatoes are still intact, about 5 minutes.

3. Remove from the heat and transfer all but a thin layer of the sauce to a bowl. Arrange 3 tortillas over the sauce in the pan, tearing and overlapping them to fit in a single layer. Spread half of the sour cream over the tortillas, then top with a third of the cheese and cilantro, then half of the beans and corn. Spread half of the remaining sauce over and top with 3 tortillas, the remaining sour cream, a third of the cheese and cilantro, and the remaining beans and corn. Top with the last 3 tortillas and the remaining sauce, cheese, and cilantro.

4. Bake until bubbly and golden, about 30 minutes. Let cool in the pan for 10 minutes before serving.

Tabbouleh
(Bulgur and Lentil Salad)

SERVES 4

1 cup bulgur

1 cup lentils, preferably French green lentils, picked over, rinsed, and drained

Salt and freshly ground black pepper

½ cup fresh lemon juice, plus lemon wedges for garnish

2 tablespoons extra-virgin olive oil

4 large tomatoes, cored, seeded, chopped

1 English (seedless) cucumber, peeled in alternating strips and chopped

1 cup packed fresh flat-leaf parsley leaves, finely chopped

1 small garlic clove, minced

1. Bring 6 cups water to a boil in a large saucepan.

2. Place the bulgur in a large heatproof bowl and add 2 cups of the boiling water. Let stand 10 minutes or until the water is absorbed and the bulgur is tender. Drain if necessary.

3. Meanwhile, generously salt the remaining boiling water and add the lentils. When the water boils again, reduce the heat to medium low and simmer until the lentils are tender, about 25 minutes. Drain well.

4. Whisk together the lemon juice and oil in a large bowl and add the bulgur, lentils, tomatoes, cucumber, parsley, and garlic. Season to taste with salt and pepper and stir well. Cover and refrigerate until cold, at least 2 hours and up to overnight.

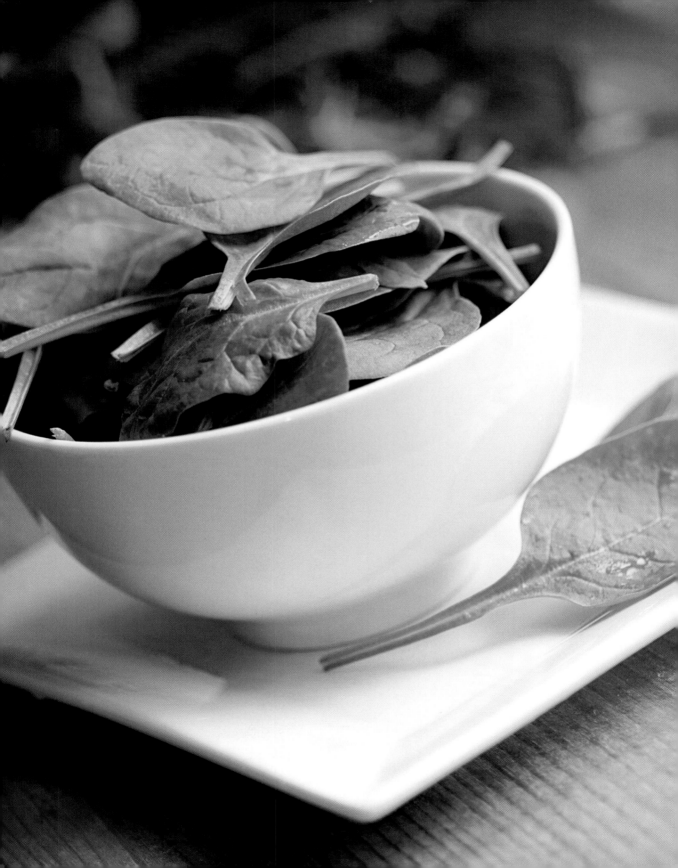

Sautéed Spinach with Garlic

SERVES 4

1 tablespoon extra-virgin
olive oil

2 garlic cloves, lightly crushed

12 ounces baby spinach

1 tablespoon chopped fresh
dill leaves

Salt and freshly ground
black pepper

1. Combine the oil and garlic in a large skillet and set over medium heat. Cook until the garlic is fragrant and golden, about 2 minutes.

2. Add the spinach and dill, season with salt and pepper, and cook, gently stirring, until just wilted, about 2 minutes.

Roasted Root Vegetables

SERVES 4

4 red potatoes, cut into 2-inch chunks

3 medium carrots, cut into 2-inch chunks

3 medium parsnips, cut into 2-inch chunks

1 fennel bulb, cut into wedges

1 medium red onion, cut into wedges

3 tablespoons olive oil

4 fresh rosemary sprigs

Salt and freshly ground black pepper

1. Preheat the oven to 400°F.

2. Combine the potatoes, carrots, parsnips, fennel, onion, oil, rosemary, and a pinch each of salt and pepper in a large rimmed baking sheet. Toss until well mixed and evenly coated. Spread in an even layer.

3. Roast, stirring once or twice, until the vegetables are browned and tender, about 1 hour. Discard rosemary.

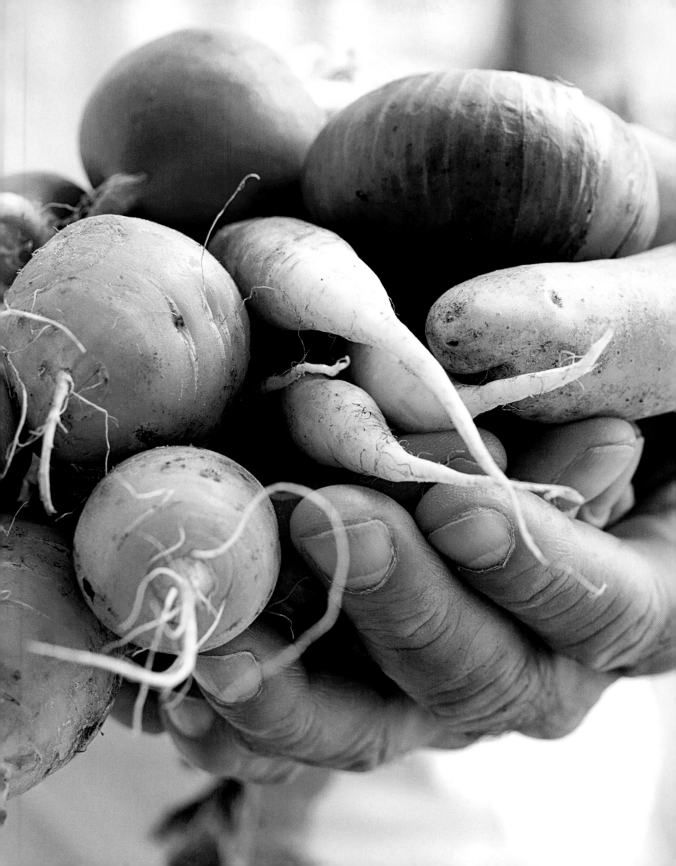

Calico
Bean Salad

SERVES 4

2 tablespoons extra-virgin olive oil

2 tablespoons fresh lime juice

2 tablespoons finely chopped fresh flat-leaf parsley leaves

2 tablespoons finely chopped fresh cilantro leaves

1 teaspoon ground cumin

Salt and freshly ground black pepper

2 cups frozen corn kernels, thawed

2 15-ounce cans black beans, rinsed and drained

1 red bell pepper, stemmed, seeded, and diced

1 green bell pepper, stemmed, seeded, and diced

2 green onions, finely chopped, optional

1. Whisk together the oil, lime juice, parsley, cilantro, and cumin in a large bowl. Season to taste with salt and pepper.

2. Add the corn, beans, peppers, and green onions. Lightly toss until evenly coated and season to taste. Cover and refrigerate for up to 2 hours before serving.

Banbury Tart

MAKES 1 LARGE TART

⅔ cup dried currants

¼ cup finely chopped citron*

½ cup sugar, plus more for topping

1 teaspoon cornstarch

1 teaspoon freshly grated lemon peel

1 tablespoon fresh lemon juice

1 14-ounce box refrigerated pre-rolled pie pastry (with 2 dough rounds)

1 tablespoon whole milk

1. Combine the currants, citron, and ⅓ cup water in a small saucepan. Bring to a boil over high heat, reduce the heat to medium, and simmer for 3 minutes.

2. Meanwhile, mix the sugar with the cornstarch in a small bowl. Add to the currant mixture and cook, stirring constantly, until the mixture is slightly thickened, about 5 minutes. Remove from the heat. Stir in the lemon peel and juice and let the mixture cool to room temperature.

3. Preheat the oven to 375°F. Line a baking sheet with parchment paper.

4. Place 1 pastry round on the prepared sheet. Spread the currant mixture over the pastry, leaving a ½-inch rim. Use a little water to dampen the rim. Center the other pastry round on top, then use a fork to press and seal the edge. Brush the top pastry with the milk and sprinkle with sugar. Cut three vents in the center of the top pastry.

5. Bake until the crust is golden and cooked through, about 30 minutes.

6. Let cool completely in the pan on a wire rack. Cut into thin wedges.

*Citron is widely available in supermarkets around the winter holidays and in specialty food stores the rest of the year.

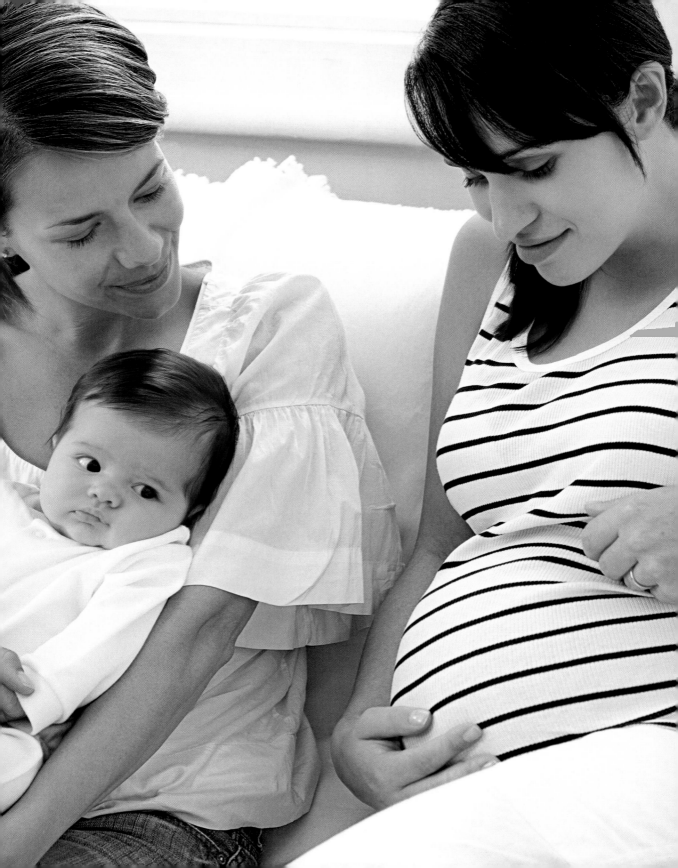

Chapter 2

Hungry Baby, Hungry Mom: The Best Foods for New Mothers

NEWBORNS TO 6 WEEKS

Sometime in the not-so-distant future, you aren't going to remember every detail of your labor. What all those veteran moms say is clichéd but true: you don't remember the pain as much as you remember the pleasure of finally holding your child for the first time. Unfortunately, if you're reading this book with your newborn sleeping—or not sleeping—in your arms or nearby, you're not in the pain-free-memories-of-labor-and-delivery zone. In fact, depending on how old (that is, new) your baby is, you are probably capable of instant recall.

If you're like most postpartum mothers, we'll assume you're still feeling a little tender here and there, but it gets better and it gets easier. We hope that you're reaching out for crucial breastfeeding support in these early days and weeks and that you've created a helping network that works for you. Beyond your partner, friends, family members, and health care providers, breastfeeding assistance and information are readily available through La Leche League International, and our active and friendly community will welcome you with mother-to-mother support, in person through our meetings, over the phone, and via our website and its many educational resources and forums. (Visit our website at www.llli.org, call our U.S.-based phone line, 877-4-LA LECHE (877-

452-5324), and see our book **The Womanly Art of Breastfeeding** for more in-depth breastfeeding help and information.)

We want to help you be successful at breastfeeding, and we know that feeding your newborn baby is one of your most important jobs as a mother right now—but who can work on an empty stomach? Baby isn't the only one who's hungry . . . let's eat!

> "The first 3 months post-partum it's essential that you get enough nutrition to allow your body to heal and to make milk. Making good nutritious and plentiful milk needs to be your main focus right now. Eat to hunger, drink to thirst, and nurse your baby tons, at least every two hours. This will set you up for a successful breastfeeding relationship."

Feeding on Demand: It's Not Just for Your Baby

During pregnancy, you probably added an additional 350 calories or so to your diet, and you should aim for the same number for the first 6 months of breastfeeding (this actually goes up slightly, to about 400 calories, after 6 months). Your body is doing a different job now—making milk rather than building a baby—and you still need those extra calories. You should also still aim to get those calories through high-quality nutrition rather than empty calories, through healthy snacks, and by supplementing your regular meals.

But when you're feeding a newborn on demand and simply getting used to being a mother (even if you've done it before, **this** baby is new), the "eat healthfully" advice is not always so easy to follow. Perhaps you've got a good supply of food on hand, but your refrigerator, freezer, and cabinets won't replenish themselves, and in the early days and weeks you won't be standing in the kitchen preparing multicourse meals or lingering over them at the dinner table.

If you have a support network, even an informal one, you will have offers of help, and hopefully they sound something like this: **Can I bring you lunch or dinner? . . . I'm dropping off a hot meal. . . . What do you need from the grocery store? . . . I baked you a dozen bran muffins—and my amazing brownies. . . . I can stop and get take-out on the way home from work, whatever you're craving. . . . We made my grandma's chicken soup and froze some**

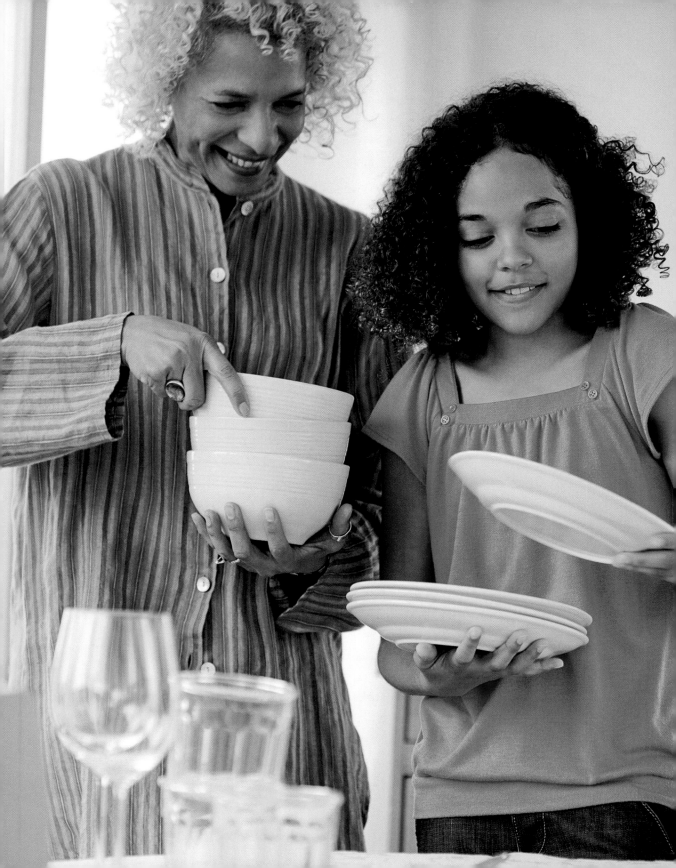

extra for you. If you are lucky enough to have offers like those, say yes to all of them! Better yet, learn to take these offers of help and turn them into food that's really good for you—and your baby, too.

When someone asks, "What do you need?" and "What do you want to eat?" be ready to direct them with specific, nutrition-packed answers. (Don't hesitate to hand your would-be helpers the recipes in this book—such as the hearty Three-Cheese Lasagna with Italian Sausage on page 81, an LLLI Member's Favorite that offers calcium, protein, and more and has seen many a mom through the newborn phase.) Let's look at the major nutrients your body will benefit from right now, with a reminder that there are no special foods that will cause you to make more or better milk. Your goal is to stay strong and healthy as you recover from childbirth and embark on breastfeeding, and making sure you get nutrition-dense foods is key.

The chart in Chapter 1 (pages 10–11) should still serve as a guideline of sorts. Your postpartum needs for these major nutrients do not change radically (though there is an increased need for protein, as you'll see below), and their food sources remain the same—good to know if you are thinking about what to eat or how to respond to that offer of help. Here are the recommended daily intakes (the higher range) for your reference:[1]

> **PROTEIN:** An increase of 40–70 grams over basic (nonpregnant) protein needs (depending on your BMI); a breastfeeding mother may need more than 100 grams of protein a day
>
> **CALCIUM:** 1,000 milligrams
>
> **IRON:** 9 milligrams
>
> **FIBER:** 28 grams
>
> **FOLATE:** 500 micrograms. During pregnancy the recommended daily intake for folate is 600 micrograms per day, because of the developing fetal brain. Now that you are no longer pregnant, this level can drop down to about 500 micrograms; another pregnancy is probably not at the top of your to-do list right now, but should you plan to get pregnant in the future, you'll want to maintain a higher level of folate than the daily intake of 400 micrograms recommended for nonpregnant women.

As for DHA (see pages 17–18), this essential fatty acid continues to be crucial postpartum. Your baby's brain will grow rapidly during the first year of life, nearly tripling in weight by her first birthday (from about 110 grams to 350 grams). About half of the brain is made up of DHA, the omega-3 "good fat" found primarily in cold-water fish. DHA also influences the development of the eye's retina. Fortunately, your milk is rich in good fats including DHA, but consuming fish such as salmon, sardines, and tuna will ensure even higher levels of this brain builder. Postpartum moms still need the 200–300 milligrams of DHA a day recommended during pregnancy.

Though the best DHA food source is fish, there are others as well, such as fortified eggs and other fortified foods, which offer smaller amounts. Foods such as flaxseed (available in supermarkets ground or whole) and soy contain another good fat, linolenic acid, which the body can convert to DHA. However, only 0.2 percent of the linolenic acid found in flaxseed and soy can be converted to DHA, so fish truly is a superior source. (See the list of seafood recipes in this book on page 33.) There are also many popular fish oil supplements that can be purchased, though algae-derived DHA may be preferable, as it is free of potential toxins such as mercury, which can accumulate in fish fat. (Note that fish oil supplements are not regulated by the FDA.)

You Need a Few Extra Things in Your Diet Right Now—What About Your Baby?

Sunlight is the body's primary source of vitamin D, as it allows humans to manufacture their own supply of this nutrient, which promotes the absorption of calcium for bone growth and health and keeps our immune system strong. But many inhabitants of northern or rainy climates find it hard to get the sun exposure they need for vitamin D production. Also, in recent years people have been warned about the thinning ozone layer and the resulting dangers of skin cancer; the preventive use of sunscreen is now so prevalent that many experts worry we do not receive enough vitamin D from sunlight. As a result, many public health groups suggest

---

**You Need a Few Extra Things in Your Diet
Right Now—What About Your Baby?** (CONTINUED)

that most of us—even exclusively breastfed babies—need additional vitamin D from supplements.

Many pediatricians recommend giving all newborns a vitamin D supplement (400 IU per day) for the first year of life, to prevent bone-weakening rickets. Alternatively, as we suggest in **The Womanly Art of Breastfeeding**, you can talk to your doctor about increasing the level of vitamin D in your milk by taking a vitamin D supplement yourself. There is research to suggest that 4,000 IU per day may be the amount needed to get an adequate level into your milk.

There are safe ways to expose your baby to the sun, just by going in and out of the house to get the mail or run errands. These brief but effective exposures to sunlight will assist with vitamin D production. (Use sunscreen sparingly until your baby is 6 months old, and then only if his sun exposure will be prolonged.) As we suggest in **The Womanly Art of Breastfeeding**, which contains additional information on ways to help your baby get vitamin D, discuss with your doctor to see if your baby needs supplementation. You can find drops that are only vitamin D, put the drops on your nipple, and let the baby nurse them off. ■

Not Just What to Eat but How

You don't need to be convinced to eat—assuming you're starting to feel you're your old self, your new work is giving you a healthy appetite. But how can you nourish your baby and nourish your body at the same time, particularly when you only have one hand free and few opportunities to sit, undisturbed, for a regular meal? Another thing to consider: if you are on maternity leave or are home alone at least during the workday, **you** are the only grown-up you need to feed. (If you have a toddler, preschooler, or school-age kids to keep you company, see Chapter 5 for some ideas for older kids' snacks and meals.) You won't

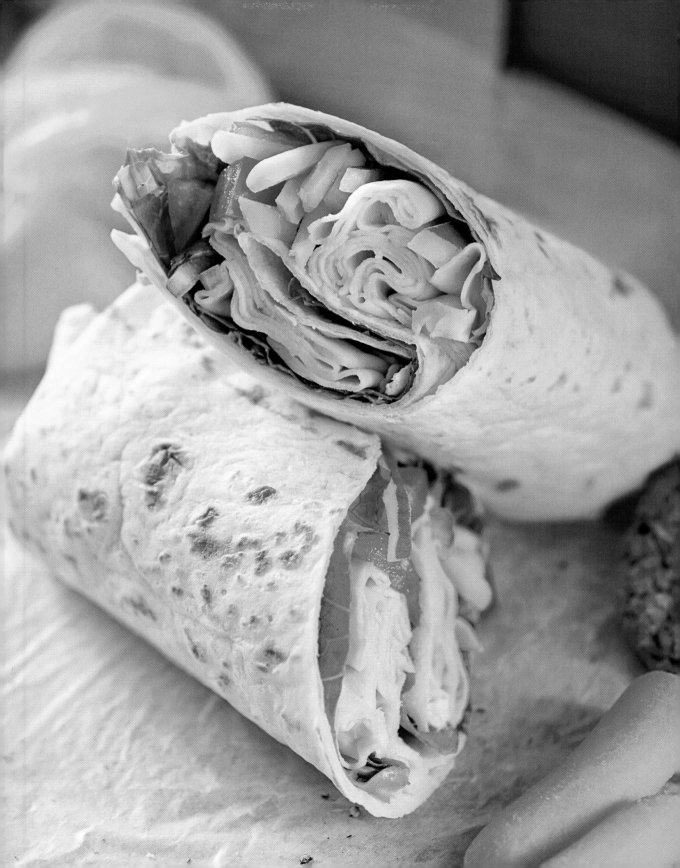

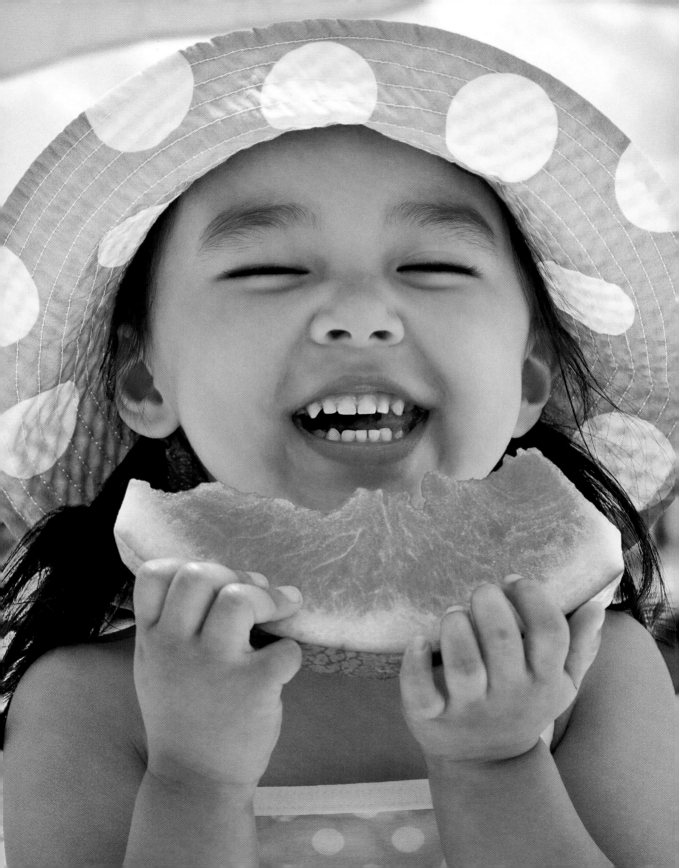

want to spend a lot of time in the kitchen making a meal for one, which is all the more reason to tap into your own personal Food Network and let friends and family bring you foods you can refrigerate or freeze in single-serve portions, to be reheated as needed.

Here are some of our favorite ideas for quick and easy meals and snacks that you can enjoy without putting your baby down, whether you are wearing him, nursing her, or just snuggling together. Think of these as finger foods for grown-ups, no utensils necessary. While you can make many of them yourself, you can also buy items such as presliced fruits or veggies or high-quality hummus (again, read the labels) at many grocery stores. You may not be used to shopping for these convenience foods, but in many cases it's worth the time you'll save. Better yet, when that person in your support network offers help, put these items on your shopping list and hand it off. (Don't forget to look back at Chapter 1; many of our quick-and-easy pregnancy snack and meal ideas will work postpartum, too.)

FOODS YOU CAN EAT WITH ONE HAND

- **Wraps, pitas, and sandwiches.** We like pitas and other pocket breads best because they are self-contained (no tomato slices sliding out onto baby's head) and just about crumb-free. Fill as you wish—lean turkey, calcium-packed cheeses, and fiber-rich vegetables are best picks. (Add a side of baked pita chips or whole-grain pretzels, some fruit, and a glass of low-fat milk or other dairy and you've got a one-handed lunch.)
- **Presliced vegetables.** Try carrots, bell peppers, and celery with healthy dips. Try hummus, tahini, or Greek tzatziki (yogurt-cucumber dip).
- **Think easy-to-eat fruit.** Apples, cantaloupe cubes, bananas, grapes, and berries are all good, as are orange slices (peel before you get comfortable).
- **Baked goods to go.** Choose whole-grain muffins and bagels, slices of multigrain bread, quick breads, and whole-grain cookies. (See our LLLI Member's Favorite recipes at the end of this chapter for Banana-Nut Bread and Oatmeal Raisin Cookies.)
- **Smoothies.** Break out the blender and start with low-fat yogurt (the thick

"Make your own trail mix and keep it in your diaper bag. I couldn't eat nuts, so I made great trail mix with pumpkin seeds and dried fruit. If you eat dairy, cheese sticks are great. Hummus and veggies—those little carrots are great—because fiber in veggies slows down the absorption of sugar so the food will last a bit longer and stabilize your blood sugar. And sandwiches, sandwiches, sandwiches! I always have a giant vat of tuna salad around that I can throw on bread—I funk up tuna with cranberries and curry powder. Chicken salad with cranberries and tarragon is good, too, and easy. And I keep a few frozen dinners for emergencies."

Greek-style variety is highest in protein) and the fruit of your choice. Add ice if desired, thin with skim milk, and give it an omega-3 kick with a tablespoon of ground flaxseed. (See our Super Smoothie with Yogurt, Berries, and Bananas recipe at the end of this chapter.) Once you get the hang of it, making smoothies and customizing them for your tastes is simple.

- **"Bar" food.** High-quality granola or energy bars, that is. (Read the labels!)
- **An ice cream cone.** Go ahead, you deserve it.

At some point you'll feel pretty confident about simultaneously feeding your baby and eating, but your newly acquired one-handed skills have limits. Here are some commonsense reminders from multitasking moms who have nursed, nibbled, and sipped simultaneously:

- Avoid drinking hot beverages or handling overflowing cups and glasses.
- Careful with those utensils—finger foods are best for quick meals or snacks so you don't have to fumble with forks and knives in close proximity to baby's head and body. (Eat that yogurt with a plastic spoon: the container won't tip over, and if you drop the spoon, no harm done that you can't wipe away.)
- Skip the soup (save it for sitting at the table) unless it's chilled and you're sipping it.
- Think twice if you're eating something messy, sloshy, drippy, or slippery—your nursling can handle a few crumbs raining down here and there but probably will object to a vinaigrette shower or a hat made out of pizza toppings.
- If you generally nurse in the same spot, turn the nightstand or end table into your personal dining table. Clear off the clutter, put down a tray or

place mat, keep napkins and wipes handy, and you've got a satellite dining room. (And more than one mom has installed a mini-fridge in her nursling's room!)

Just Eat: When and Where Don't Matter

As we pointed out in **The Womanly Art of Breastfeeding**, and as generations of mothers will tell you, life won't be like this forever, but it is for now. You won't always eat finger foods with one hand, and you won't always be dining in rooms, on furniture, and in positions that you don't usually use for eating. You won't always make a meal out of a glass of milk and a quick PB&J eaten at the kitchen counter between feedings, or hope that someone will swing by with tonight's dinner in exchange for a look at the new baby. You won't always be eating breakfast at five in the morning or lunch at three in the afternoon. You won't be worrying about how you'll manage a trip to the store with a newborn, or what to buy when you get there.

You will have time for preparing and enjoying your favorite foods again. You will, at some point very soon, return to the table, sit at your place (with nothing and no one in your lap but a napkin), and enjoy a "normal" meal—whether that involves good wine and adult conversation, a chance to eat a turkey sandwich

"For many breastfeeding mothers, knowing what to eat is not nearly as challenging as finding the time for shopping and cooking. But good nutrition doesn't mean spending more time in the kitchen. Many foods are both nutritious and handy for snacking and quick meals. Cheese, yogurt, whole-grain bread or crackers, tomatoes, sprouts, fresh fruits, whole or sliced raw vegetables, hard-cooked eggs, and nuts can be eaten with little or no preparation. More frequent smaller meals can be just as nutritious as three larger meals. Rather than preparing three large meals a day, some nursing mothers try to have a healthy snack and something to drink every time they sit down to nurse."

—FROM LA LECHE LEAGUE INTERNATIONAL'S *THE BREASTFEEDING ANSWER BOOK*[2]

and chips without interruption, or a quiet morning with coffee, toast, and the newspaper. You will use the table manners your mother taught you, which you will in turn teach your child. But not now.

Instead, this newborn nursling is your new reality—and this phase is exceedingly brief. Good food gives you much-needed energy and helps you maintain your milk supply. You need energy, and your baby needs milk. So eat—however and whenever you choose to do so—for your own well-being and for that of your child. Your place at the table will be waiting.

I Like It—but Does My Baby Want to Eat the Same Thing?

It was true before your baby was born and it's still the case: she's eating what you're eating. But does she enjoy the garlicky taste of your family's spaghetti sauce as much as you do? What about those fragrantly spiced homemade tamales your partner's tía dropped off? You were practically raised on your Louisiana grandmother's red beans and rice, and your sister just brought over a batch, but beans . . . won't there be gassy consequences for your baby?

Unless you truly suspect your baby has a serious food sensitivity or allergy, don't hesitate to continue to eat the good, wholesome foods you've always eaten. If you come from a family or background where special dishes, spices, and ingredients are a prized part of your heritage, they are part of your baby's heritage, too. You are passing along your culture through your milk, and if it tastes like onions, so be it. It's true that what you eat will affect the taste of your milk, but—unless it's truly distressing your nursling (see "Food Sensitivities and Allergies" on pages 126–28)—that should not be a concern. All over the world, women from many different cultures are eating wildly divergent diets and nursing their healthy, thriving babies. From India to Italy to Idaho, the milk these mothers produce is as different in taste as the foods they eat, but the result is the same: well-nourished children, wherever they are.

And if you are wondering if there will be gassy consequences for baby should you eat the Minestrone with White Beans and Loads of Vegetables (see recipe page 85), there is really only one way to find out!

Adorable but Gassy . . . Was It Something I Ate?

If you're concerned about the connection between what you're eating and your newborn's gassy symphony, remember that babies have no inhibitions when it comes to letting loose, and that broccoli you ate may have nothing to do with the normal levels of intestinal gas that build up in his tiny tummy.

Gas is normal. If gas seems excessive and your nursling is uncomfortable, check in with your pediatrician or a lactation expert. Your baby may be getting too much milk (her tiny tummy holds only about 3 ounces right now), or you may need to try some different ways, beyond burping, to help her avoid gas buildup, such as holding her upright against your chest and shoulders to stimulate release of the bubbles.

If your baby's gassiness really concerns you, try keeping a food diary to see if you can connect your baby's gassy spells to what you've consumed, and then, of course, eat less of the food that affects her digestion. But remember, if the gas is not causing your baby discomfort or interfering with breastfeeding, don't spend a lot of time playing toot detective. This too shall . . . pass.

Are You Eating Your Vegetables? (Fruits, Too!)

When friends offer to take your order for lunch or dinner, ask them to include a big garden salad, plenty of vegetables, and some fresh fruit. These may not sound as tempting as freshly baked chocolate chip cookies (your friends can bring some of those, too), and when you're sleep-deprived and trying to put together a meal, nutrient-packed vegetables might not rank high on your menu. However, they remain an important food source for you and your nursling, and you should aim for a minimum of three to five servings of vegetables per day. One serving typically equals 1 cup of leafy vegetables, ½ cup of cooked or raw vegetables, or ¾ cup of pure vegetable juice. We've given you plenty of veggie side dish recipes in this book, such as Celery Root and Potato Puree, Orange-

Braised Baby Carrots, and Roasted Beets with Balsamic Dressing (pages 187, 186, and 236). Vegetable-packed recipes such as our Summer Squash Omelets on page 180 can be served as a main dish.

As you know by now, nearly all fruits and vegetables are low-calorie, nutritionally dense food sources. During pregnancy and breastfeeding, your body requires more fluids, increased amounts of certain vitamins and minerals, and more energy-making calories. By upping the amount of fruits and veggies on your plate, you'll meet all these needs. They provide hydration, have loads of useful nutrients, reduce the risks of certain illnesses, can be an excellent source of fiber, and truly are the ultimate convenience food—fresh, frozen, or canned.

When you can, shop seasonally for fresh produce. Consider joining a Community Supported Agriculture organization (a CSA), where for a fee members can "subscribe" to a delivery of superfresh, locally grown seasonal produce from area farmers. It's like the local farmer's market coming to you! Depending on how much produce a CSA delivers during the growing season, you may even want to share a membership with another family. (Generally, you will agree to take delivery of whatever is in season. Families can benefit from sharing so that no one household is overwhelmed by a bushel of eggplant!) To find a CSA in your area, visit www.localharvest.org. (This website also allows you to search for local farmer's markets, family farms that sell direct, small dairies, producers of grass-fed meat, and other sources for whole foods and organic products.)

Keep frozen and canned items on hand for those out-of-season stretches, or for when you can't get to the store or visit the farmer's market. Nothing beats being able to reach into your freezer for fiber-rich, protein-packed, vitamin-filled green peas to complete a dinner, or open a can of vitamin-C-loaded tomatoes to make your favorite sauce, soup, or stew. Whole fruits and vegetables offer the most fiber and nutrients, but 100 percent juice can be healthful as well.

Look back at the chart in Chapter 1 (pages 10–11) for some fruit and vegetable sources for calcium, folate, iron, and fiber, as well as the information for zinc, magnesium, and potassium on pages 12–14, and consider the following information.[3] We'll try to highlight the less obvious sources of nutrients—

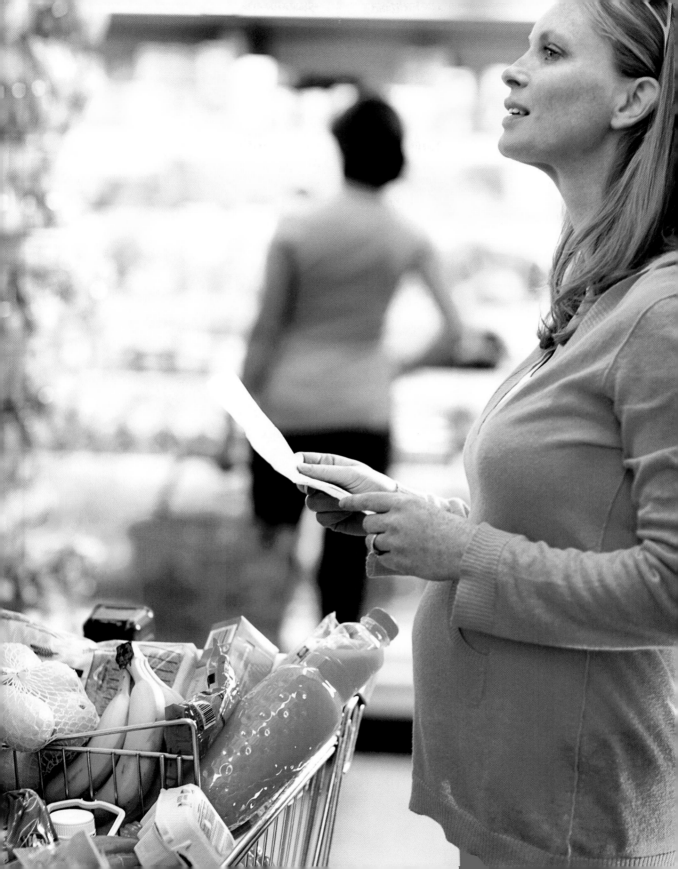

everyone knows oranges have lots of vitamin C, but did you know about ruta-baga?

If you're looking for more **fiber**: Try unpeeled apples and pears; blackberries, raisins, and raspberries; beans (lentils, pinto, lima, small white beans, and others); and spinach. Nearly all fruits and vegetables offer dietary fiber, but these are the winners for high fiber because one serving contains 5 or more grams (1 piece fruit, 1 cup berries, ½ cup beans, 1½ cups raw spinach).

If you're looking for more **vitamin C**: Beyond the mighty orange and its citrusy sisters, try apricots, berries (strawberries, raspberries, gooseberries, black-berries), guavas, papayas, melons, kiwis, pomegranates, rutabagas, collard greens, okra, onions, tomatoes—and, yes, hot chili peppers!

If you're looking for more **vitamin A**: Yellow or orange fruits and vegetables are the best source of carotene, which the body converts to vitamin A. Try car-rots, cantaloupe, peaches, nectarines, sweet potatoes, and winter squash. (Nutritionists put broccoli into this category, too, because underneath that green chlorophyll exterior it's indeed yellow!)

If you're looking for more **iron**: Winged beans (popular in Asian foods), white beans, pinto beans, lentils, spinach, and dried apricots are all great choices. (Note that while all these foods contain iron, this nutrient is best absorbed from foods containing hemoglobin, which is why red meat and poultry are usually at the top of the list.)

If you're looking for more **folate**: Consider oranges, strawberries, beans, dark green leafy veggies (spinach, collard greens, beet greens), endive, arti-chokes, or broccoli.

If you're looking for more **calcium**: Spinach, collard greens, turnip greens, calcium-fortified orange juice, soybeans (edamame), and cowpeas (black-eyed peas) are all good sources. (Note that while plant sources such as those above, as well as foods such as almonds, can provide some calcium, dairy products still offer the most absorbable forms of calcium. See pages 16–17 for more information.)

If you're looking for more **potassium**: Check out lima beans, lentils, sweet potatoes, tomatoes, bananas, cherries, and dried apricots.

If you're looking for more **magnesium**: Good sources include nuts (brazil nuts, cashews, hazelnuts, peanuts, pine nuts, walnuts), butternut squash, and many beans (especially pinto beans).

Do You Need to Go Organic?

If you are ingesting pesticides along with your strawberries, then your nursling is ingesting them, too. The levels are low enough to comply with government regulations and you are probably not endangering yourself or your child by eating an imported grape out of season; still, these are chemicals you and your baby probably don't want and definitely don't need. Practically speaking, though, the last thing you're about to do right now is head into the garden to plant your own pesticide-free carrots, and shopping for organic produce can be expensive (though in recent years, as demand has grown, prices have become more reasonable). In the short term, it's helpful to know which fruits and vegetables are safest when it comes to pesticides.

The Environmental Working Group (www.foodnews.org), a nonprofit organization dedicated to public health and consumer education, offers a useful and enlightening shopper's guide to fruits and vegetables (now available as a free downloadable app). Their Clean 15 list includes conventionally grown produce items that have the lowest levels of pesticides, while items with the highest levels of pesticides are on their Dirty Dozen list. EWG recommends that you go organic for items in the Dirty Dozen. Check EWG's website for annual updates and for detailed information on how they compile their listings.

THE CLEAN 15

Onions	Sweet peas	Cantaloupe
Avocado	Asparagus	Watermelon
Sweet corn	Kiwi	Grapefruit
Pineapple	Cabbage	Sweet potato
Mangos	Eggplant	Honeydew melon

THE DIRTY DOZEN

Celery	Blueberries	Cherries
Peaches	Nectarines	Kale/collard greens
Strawberries	Bell peppers	Potatoes
Apples	Spinach	Grapes (imported)

It goes without saying—but we'll remind you anyway—to thoroughly wash all fruits and vegetables you consume. The peel of apples and pears is rich in fiber, so eat the skin—but wash it well.

There has been extensive research done on contaminants (including pesticide residues such as DDT, PCBs, and other substances) occasionally found in human breast milk. The conclusion is that the benefits of breastfeeding generally outweigh the risks of passing on harmful levels of pesticides and other substances.[4]

Should You Still Be Taking a Prenatal Supplement?

If you took a prenatal vitamin during pregnancy, your health care provider may recommend that you continue to do so after you give birth and begin breastfeeding. This is because when you first start to breastfeed, a prenatal supplement will be helpful in replenishing your body with any nutrients that may have dipped during pregnancy. Later, during your baby's first year, you might consider a women's vitamin-mineral supplement, as you will not need as much iron as most prenatal supplements contain. When exclusively breastfeeding, during the first 6 months you probably will not be menstruating and therefore you will not lose iron from your body.

Food Is Important—but Don't Forget the Fluids

First of all, increasing the amount of fluid you drink will **not** increase your milk supply. In fact, studies show that increasing **or** decreasing fluid intake does not alter the amount of milk produced. Only in cases of **extreme** dehydration—for instance, in countries where famine is widespread or in impoverished regions where the water supply is extremely limited—will milk supply decline.

Still, if you don't drink enough water or other healthful fluids and you're breastfeeding frequently, you will feel thirsty—really, really thirsty. As one mother posted on our website, "I can chug an 8-ounce glass of water and then do it again immediately after. I still wake up and drink water at night, too!"

There is no perfect amount of water you should be drinking each day. The old eight-glasses-a-day cliché is just that. Our advice is simple: **drink to thirst**. Try keeping a refillable water bottle nearby when you nurse and sip from it as needed.[5] Have a glass of water with meals or snacks. Keep water on your nightstand. Put a water bottle in your diaper bag or stroller. If you wake up thirsty and you're nursing at night, a drink of water will be like heaven. (You may be thinking heaven is not having to wake up every few hours, but quenching your thirst ranks right up there.)

Tap water, bottled, filtered? It depends on your local water supply. Bottled water does not contain fluoride, which you need to prevent tooth decay. (Cavities aren't just for kids.) Find out if your local water supply is fluoridated; most are, but levels vary from community to community. Normal levels of fluoride in the water you drink will not harm your nursling. (In fact, your baby needs the fluoride in your milk for her developing teeth.)

If you live in an older home with lead pipes, have your water tested and use a water filter on your tap if necessary. A diet that is high in calcium, iron, and zinc can decrease absorption of lead should it get into your system. (If you're following the diet recommendations in **Feed Yourself, Feed Your Family**, you should be getting plenty of those lead-reducing nutrients.)

Water isn't your only option for hydration, but with zero calories it's one of the healthiest. Low-fat or skim milk and pure fruit juice can be healthful options, and if you're in search of nondairy calcium sources, many orange juices are now available with as much calcium per serving as milk. (Other nondairy drinkable calcium sources are fortified rice, soy, and almond milks.)

Caffeinated coffee is okay, but be aware of the amounts you consume, especially in these early days and weeks. Excessive caffeine intake can cause your baby to be wakeful, fussy, and jittery. Furthermore, you won't be able to rest or sleep, either! Caffeine will stay in your system for as much as 4 to 6 hours, so keep that in mind when you have your morning cup (avoid nursing immediately after that double latte). If you totally eliminated caffeine from your diet and are just now reintroducing it, it may have a greater impact on your baby. Try to stick to moderate levels (200 milligrams per day, about the amount in two 8-ounce cups—but check your brand; some gourmet coffees are much higher in caffeine).

Obviously, caffeine is not limited to coffee; teas, sodas, sports drinks, and other beverages can contain caffeine as well, but generally coffee packs the biggest punch. Avoid sodas with their empty calories, sugar, and caffeine—you have better ways to quench your thirst. Also note that caffeine will increase the amount of calcium excreted in your urine and result in a loss of calcium from both your breast milk and your bones.

Can I Have a Drink Now?

Yes.

Alcohol consumption is safe in moderation (for women, generally a maximum of seven drinks per week), so have that margarita you've been wanting for the last 9 months.* However, keep in mind that babies do not metabolize alcohol as well as adults do, and that the percentage of alcohol in your bloodstream is equivalent to the percentage in your milk.

Babies who drink breast milk containing alcohol have been shown to take less. Furthermore, alcohol can interfere with oxytocin, the hormone that stimulates let-down.

Our advice: as with caffeine (or with any foods that you are concerned about), simply pay attention to your baby's reaction. To minimize the amount of alcohol your baby consumes, nurse **before** you have a drink. Your milk will be alcohol free by the next feeding (usually within 2 to 3 hours).**

* According to the CDC, there is no precise definition of "moderate" drinking, but federal Dietary Guidelines for Americans consider moderate drinking for women to be one drink per day (two drinks per day for men).

** Newborns sometimes fall into a pattern of cluster feeding, so this 2-to-3-hour window may not be applicable if your tiny nursling is feeding round the clock.

Help Wanted: Turning Offers of Help into Plates of Food (and Clean Dishes)

Veteran moms will tell you: if someone offers to help—to hold the baby while you eat, to bring you a pizza, to unload the dishwasher—**don't say no**. If you refuse these offers, they have a way of stopping, and that includes when your spouse or partner volunteers to diaper and dress your newborn or bring you some lemonade or your older child wants to make you a tray of food. So what if the diaper is crooked or he put the baby in the blue outfit instead of the yellow one? Big deal if the lemonade needs more sugar or your five-year-old used half a jar of peanut butter on one sandwich. Not only is it the thought that counts—it's the fact that they are willing to help just when you need it most, **and** when you're really, really hungry.

Friends and family will be willing to do just about anything to get a look at a new baby. When they say, "Oh, he's adorable! Can I do anything while I'm here?" answer, "You sure can!" Besides the usual housekeeping chores, focus on food:

- Keep a shopping list for friends on the refrigerator door.
- If they offer to make you a meal, suggest a recipe.

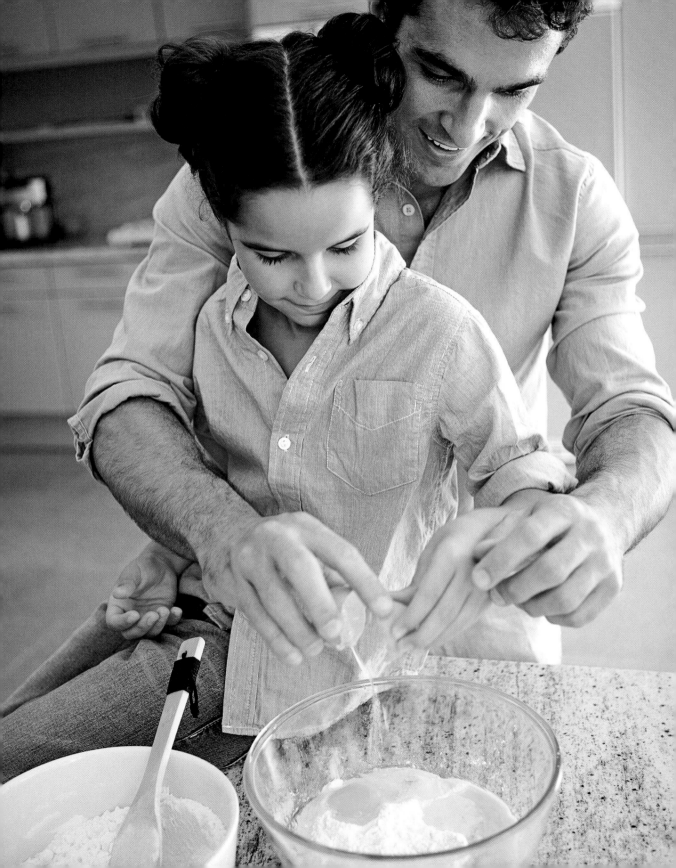

- Let them take older kids out for lunch or dinner, or make them their favorite meal.
- Let them cook for you in your kitchen (and clean up).
- If they're cooking, ask them to make a double batch of something—one for now and one for the freezer. (See the list of freezer-friendly recipes below.)
- When they're over for a visit, ask them to help you prep some snacks and mini-meals—wash and chop fresh fruits and vegetables, make up sandwiches or wraps, whip up a batch of smoothies or low-fat yogurt dips.

If you have other children, depending on their ages, let them help out with food, too—with the assistance and supervision of their dad or another adult, they can put together their own meals, and make food for you, too. If you discourage them from helping out now, they may not be so willing to offer down the road. By helping to prepare food for the family, they will feel good knowing they are contributing to the well-being of their new sibling (and Mom, too).

So just say yes when someone wants to help. And someday soon you can return the favor. There's a new mom out there who will really appreciate it.

❄ Freezer-Friendly Recipes

- ☐ Apple Bran Muffins, page 146
- ☐ Banana-Nut Bread, page 99
- ☐ Carrot-Zucchini Bread, page 239
- ☐ Chicken, Carrot, and Potato Mild Curry, page 38
- ☐ Coriander Butternut Squash Soup, page 184
- ☐ Froehlich Family's Rice, page 137
- ☐ Greek Meatballs with Yogurt Dipping Sauce (meatballs only), page 89
- ☐ Homemade Apple-Pear Sauce, page 190
- ☐ La Leche League Baking Mix, page 97 (and muffins, pancakes, or waffles made with it—pages 98, 234, and 233)
- ☐ Minted Pea Puree, page 189

Freezer-Friendly Recipes (CONTINUED)

"One of the wonderful things that our family has enjoyed with the birth of each baby is the supply of meals that friends and family have lovingly brought to our home to help us during the early weeks. Instead of fretting about coming up with something for the evening's meal, we dined on lasagna and salad as I learned to breastfeed my firstborn. . . . Each meal was delicious and, coming from different kitchens, they didn't taste like repeats. I decided to continue this delicious precedent we had enjoyed by providing a meal for others when they welcomed a baby into their family. . . . It was fun to plan and deliver a meal that would make my friend's day easier and also promote healing in her body following her baby's birth. One of the things I love about LLL is the mother-to-mother support. Providing a meal to a family with a new baby is just one practical way I delight in being able to support a fellow mother."

—RUTHIE[6]

Three-Cheese Lasagna with Italian Sausage

SERVES 12

Tomato Sauce

2 tablespoons extra-virgin olive oil

2 cups chopped onion

¼ cup finely chopped garlic

1 pound lean ground beef

12 ounces sweet or hot Italian sausage, casings removed

2 28-ounce cans crushed tomatoes in puree

½ cup tomato paste

½ cup chopped fresh basil leaves

2 tablespoons dried oregano

1 tablespoon packed light brown sugar

1 tablespoon cider or balsamic vinegar

2 dried bay leaves

½ teaspoon crushed red pepper flakes, optional

Lasagna

2 15-ounce containers part-skim ricotta cheese

½ cup freshly grated Parmesan cheese

½ cup freshly grated Pecorino Romano

1 10-ounce package frozen chopped spinach, thawed, drained, and squeezed dry

Kosher salt and freshly ground black pepper

2 large eggs

16 no-boil lasagna noodles (about 9 ounces)

5 cups freshly grated mozzarella cheese (about 1¼ pounds)

1. To make the sauce, heat the oil in a large, heavy saucepan over medium heat. Add the onion and garlic and cook, stirring occasionally, until softened, about 6 minutes.

2. Add the beef and sausage and cook, breaking the meat into small pieces with a wooden spoon, until browned, about 5 minutes.

(CONTINUED)

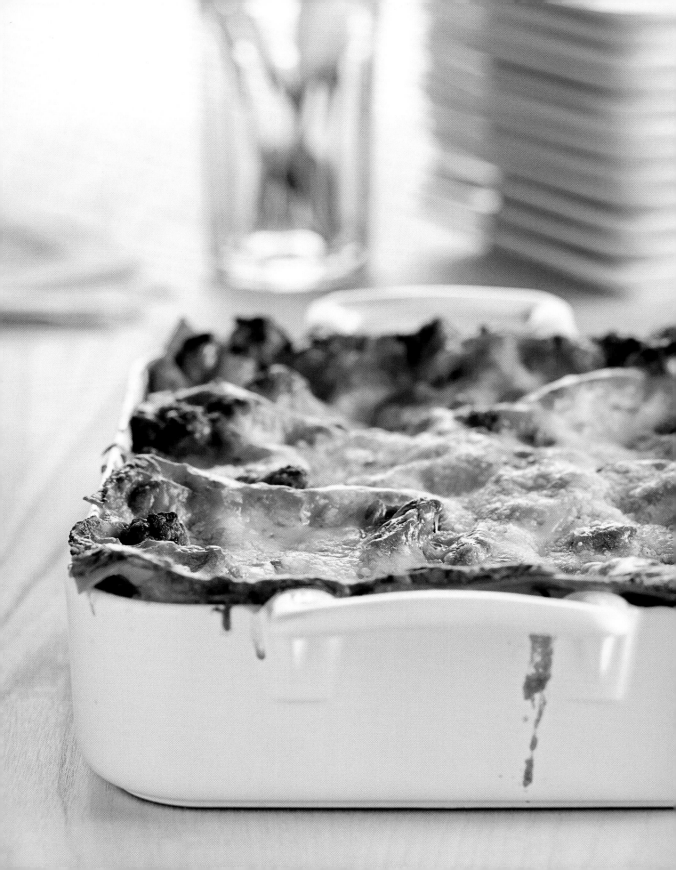

Three-Cheese Lasagna with Italian Sausage

(CONTINUED)

Note: If you do not have a 3-inch-deep baking dish, use two smaller (8-by-11-by-2-inch) baking dishes instead. Divide the fillings between the dishes, using half of the quantities above for each layer in each dish. The lasagnas can be assembled, covered, and refrigerated up to 1 day ahead. Baking times remain the same.

3. Add the crushed tomatoes, tomato paste, basil, oregano, brown sugar, vinegar, bay leaves, and pepper flakes. Cover partially, reduce the heat to medium low, and simmer, stirring occasionally, until the sauce measures about 10 cups, approximately 25 minutes. Discard the bay leaves and remove the sauce from the heat.

4. Preheat the oven to 350°F.

5. To assemble the lasagna, combine the ricotta and half of the Parmesan and Pecorino Romano in a large bowl. Stir in the spinach. Season with a pinch each of salt and pepper, then stir in the eggs until well blended.

6. Spread 1 cup of the tomato sauce in a 13-by-9-by-3-inch baking dish to cover the bottom. Arrange 5 noodles in a single layer over the sauce, overlapping to fit if necessary. Spread half of the ricotta mixture over the noodles, then sprinkle 2 cups mozzarella evenly over the ricotta mixture. Spread 3 cups sauce over the cheese. Repeat layering with 6 noodles, remaining ricotta mixture, 2 cups mozzarella, and 3 cups sauce. Arrange remaining 5 noodles over the sauce. Spread remaining sauce over the noodles, and sprinkle the remaining 1 cup mozzarella, ¼ cup Parmesan, and ¼ cup Pecorino Romano evenly over the sauce. The lasagna can be assembled, covered, and refrigerated up to 1 day ahead.

7. Cover the baking dish tightly with foil. Bake for 40 minutes, then uncover and bake until hot and bubbly, about 40 minutes. Let the lasagna stand for 15 minutes before serving.

Slow Cooker Spinach Lasagna

SERVES 12

2 10-ounce packages frozen chopped spinach, thawed, drained, and squeezed dry

2 pounds part-skim ricotta cheese

½ cup shredded Parmesan cheese

2 large eggs, lightly beaten

1 teaspoon dried oregano

½ teaspoon dried marjoram

2 25-ounce jars pasta sauce

1 package no-cook lasagna noodles

4 cups shredded mozzarella cheese

1. Mix the spinach, ricotta, Parmesan, eggs, oregano, and marjoram in a large bowl.

2. Spread one-quarter of the pasta sauce over the bottom of a 5½-quart slow cooker. Top with a layer of noodles, breaking the pieces to fit. Spread half of the spinach mixture evenly over the noodles and sprinkle with one-third of the mozzarella. Repeat the sauce, noodle, spinach, and mozzarella layering one more time. Spread half of the remaining sauce on top of the mozzarella, top with a final layer of noodles, and finish with the remaining sauce and mozzarella.

3. Cover and cook on the low setting for 7 hours or on the high setting for 4 hours. It is done when the noodles are tender, the cheese on top melted and bubbling, and the lasagna hot throughout.

Minestrone with White Beans and Loads of Vegetables

SERVES 4

2 tablespoons extra-virgin olive oil

2 large carrots, diced

2 large celery stalks, diced

1 medium onion, diced

2 garlic cloves, finely chopped

2 medium sweet potatoes, peeled and diced

8 cups lower-sodium vegetable broth

¼ teaspoon dried oregano

Salt and freshly ground black pepper

1 15-ounce can white kidney beans (cannellini), drained and rinsed

8 ounces green beans, trimmed and cut into 1-inch pieces

½ cup alphabet or other small pasta, such as ditalini

1 pound Swiss chard, tough stems cut out and discarded, leaves chopped

6 ounces baby spinach

Zest of 1 lemon

½ cup freshly grated Pecorino Romano or Parmesan cheese

1. Heat the oil in a large, heavy saucepan over medium heat. Add the carrots, celery, and onion and cook, stirring occasionally, until the vegetables are lightly browned and just tender, about 10 minutes. Stir in the garlic and cook for 1 minute.

2. Add the sweet potatoes, broth, oregano, and a pinch each of salt and pepper. Bring to a boil over high heat, then reduce the heat to medium low, cover, and simmer until a knife pierces easily through the potatoes, about 10 minutes.

3. Add the white beans, green beans, and pasta. Bring to a boil, then cook, stirring occasionally, until the green beans and pasta are just tender, about 5 minutes. Stir in the Swiss chard, spinach, and lemon zest. Cook just until the greens wilt, about 3 minutes. (The soup can be refrigerated in an airtight container overnight and reheated.)

4. Divide the hot soup among bowls and top with the cheese.

Avgolemono

SERVES 6

1 whole (3½-pound) chicken

1 carrot, chopped

1 celery stalk, chopped

1 medium onion, chopped

1 tablespoon black peppercorns

Salt

1 cup long-grain white rice

3 large eggs

⅓ cup fresh lemon juice

1. Place the chicken, carrot, celery, onion, peppercorns, and a generous pinch of salt in a large pot and cover with cold water. Bring to a boil over high heat, skimming any foam that rises to the surface. Reduce the heat to medium low, cover, and simmer for 2 hours.

2. Carefully transfer the chicken to a large bowl. Strain the broth through a fine-mesh sieve into a very large bowl. Skim any fat that rises to the surface of the broth. Return the broth to the pot.

3. Bring the strained broth and rice to a boil over high heat. Reduce the heat to low, cover, and cook until the rice is tender, about 30 minutes.

4. Meanwhile, remove and discard the chicken skin and bones. Shred the chicken meat and add to the cooked rice and broth.

5. Beat the eggs in a large bowl. Continue beating while adding the lemon juice in a slow, steady stream. Continue beating while adding 2 cups of the hot broth in a slow, steady stream. Stir the egg mixture into the broth. Continue simmering until the broth has thickened slightly, about 5 minutes.

Avgolemono: A Mother Remembers

My oldest daughter is severely allergic to milk. We discovered this allergy just as she entered her teen years, and it meant many adjustments for her. Most teenage activities include food—cheesy, milky food! Think of pizza and donuts and tacos and ice cream and all the hidden milk in most of the foods we eat. It was difficult for her to be different from everyone else, to draw attention to her special needs, and to do without some of her favorite meals. We were so happy to discover avgolemono (Greek Chicken and Rice Soup with Lemon) because it fulfilled her desire for a thick, rich, creamy soup without exposing her to milk at all! Beaten eggs thicken the soup and produce a delicious, creamy, comfort food that even now, at 25 years old, she will call and ask me to make for her on a stressful day.

—JUANA

Chicken and Sugar Snap Pea Sauté

SERVES 4

1 pound boneless, skinless chicken breasts, cut into ½-inch chunks

Salt and freshly ground black pepper

3 tablespoons extra-virgin olive oil

2 red bell peppers, stemmed, seeded, and diced

1 garlic clove, finely chopped

8 ounces sugar snap peas

1 tablespoon balsamic vinegar

2 tablespoons chopped fresh basil leaves

1. Season the chicken with salt and pepper.

2. Heat 2 tablespoons oil in a large skillet over medium-high heat. Add the chicken in a single layer and cook until browned, about 2 minutes. Turn the pieces over and cook until browned and the inside of the meat just loses its pink color, about 2 minutes. Transfer to a dish.

3. Heat the remaining tablespoon oil in the same skillet over medium heat. Add the peppers and garlic and cook, stirring occasionally, until just tender, about 5 minutes. Add the snap peas, 3 tablespoons water, and a pinch each of salt and pepper and cook, stirring occasionally, until the peas are bright green and crisp-tender, about 4 minutes.

4. Stir the chicken into the mixture, along with the vinegar and basil, and cook 1 minute more. Season to taste with salt and pepper.

Greek Meatballs with Yogurt Dipping Sauce

SERVES 4

2 tablespoons extra-virgin olive oil

2 slices whole-wheat bread

1 pound ground turkey

2 green onions, finely chopped

1 large egg

1 teaspoon ground cumin

Salt and freshly ground black pepper

1 English (seedless) cucumber, scrubbed well and diced

2 cups nonfat plain yogurt

2 tablespoons chopped fresh mint leaves

1 garlic clove, minced, optional

Whole-wheat pita breads, toasted, optional

1. Preheat the oven to 450°F. Line a large rimmed baking sheet with foil and lightly grease the foil with 1 tablespoon oil.

2. Pulse the bread in a food processor to form fine crumbs. Transfer to a large bowl and add the turkey, onion, egg, cumin, and a pinch each of salt and pepper. Use your hands to combine the ingredients until well mixed, then form the mixture into 1-inch meatballs. Wet your hands to make the shaping easier.

3. Transfer the meatballs to the prepared pan. Lightly brush the remaining tablespoon of oil on the tops of the meatballs.

4. Roast until the meat is cooked through, about 15 minutes.

5. Meanwhile, combine the cucumber, yogurt, mint, and garlic in a medium bowl until well mixed. Season to taste with salt and pepper. Serve with the meatballs and pitas.

Whole-Wheat Spaghetti with Anchovies and Cauliflower

SERVES 4

3 tablespoons extra-virgin olive oil

1 large onion, finely chopped

1 pound cauliflower florets, chopped

1 2-ounce can anchovies, rinsed and patted dry

¼ cup pitted Kalamata olives, rinsed, drained, and chopped

1 14-ounce box whole-wheat spaghetti

2 tablespoons chopped fresh basil leaves

Freshly ground black pepper

1. Bring a large pot of water to a boil.

2. Meanwhile, heat the oil in a large skillet over medium heat. Add the onion and cook, stirring occasionally, until tender and golden, about 7 minutes.

3. Add the cauliflower and ¼ cup water and cook, stirring occasionally, until the water evaporates and the cauliflower is golden brown and tender, about 7 minutes. Add the anchovies and olives and cook, stirring and breaking up the anchovies into small pieces, until well combined and fragrant, about 1 minute.

4. Meanwhile, cook the spaghetti according to the package directions. Reserve ½ cup pasta cooking liquid, then drain the spaghetti and return it to the pot. Add the cauliflower mixture, basil, and a pinch of pepper. Toss until well mixed, adding reserved water if the mixture is dry.

Crab Tostadas

SERVES 8

4 limes

1 pound fresh cooked lump crabmeat, picked over for bits of shell

1 tablespoon extra-virgin olive oil

2 tablespoons mayonnaise

3 tablespoons finely chopped red or green onion

3 plum tomatoes, cored, seeded, and chopped

1 avocado, pitted, peeled, and diced

¼ cup chopped fresh cilantro leaves, plus more for garnish

Salt and freshly ground black pepper

1 fresh jalapeño pepper, stemmed, seeded, and finely chopped, optional

8 tostada shells

1. Finely zest 2 limes into a large bowl, then juice the limes into the bowl. Quarter the remaining 2 limes and set aside.

2. To the lime zest and juice, add the crab, oil, mayonnaise, onion, tomatoes, avocado, and cilantro. Gently fold until well blended. Season to taste with salt and pepper.

3. Set up a make-your-own tostada bar: Place the crabmeat mixture in a serving bowl and garnish with cilantro. Place the tostada shells and lime wedges on a serving platter and the jalapeño in a small bowl.

Mounds of Mussels

SERVES 4

4 tablespoons (½ stick) unsalted butter

½ cup finely chopped onion

2 garlic cloves, finely chopped

1 tablespoon finely chopped fresh flat-leaf parsley leaves

⅛ teaspoon fresh thyme leaves, finely chopped

Kosher salt and freshly ground black pepper

1 cup dry white wine

3 pounds mussels, beards removed if necessary, cleaned well

1 loaf whole-grain French bread, sliced and toasted

1. Melt the butter in a large pot over medium-high heat. Add the onion, garlic, parsley, thyme, and a pinch each of salt and pepper. Cook, stirring occasionally, until the onion and garlic are softened, about 3 minutes.

2. Add the wine and bring to a boil. Cook until the wine has reduced by one-third, about 5 minutes. Add the mussels, cover, and cook, shaking the pan occasionally, until the shells open, about 8 minutes. Discard any mussels that do not open.

3. Divide the mussels and all of the pan juices among bowls. Serve with the bread for dunking.

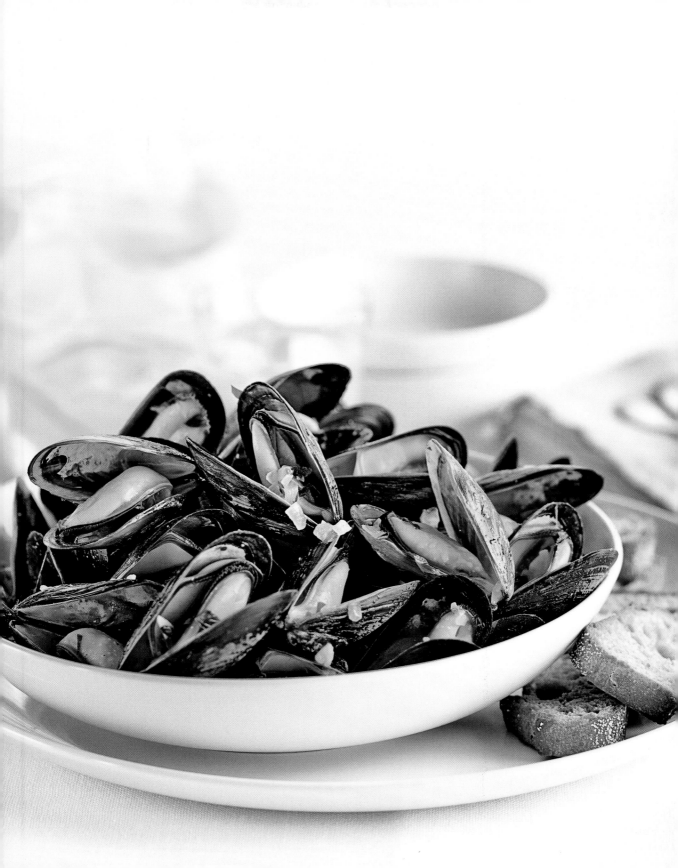

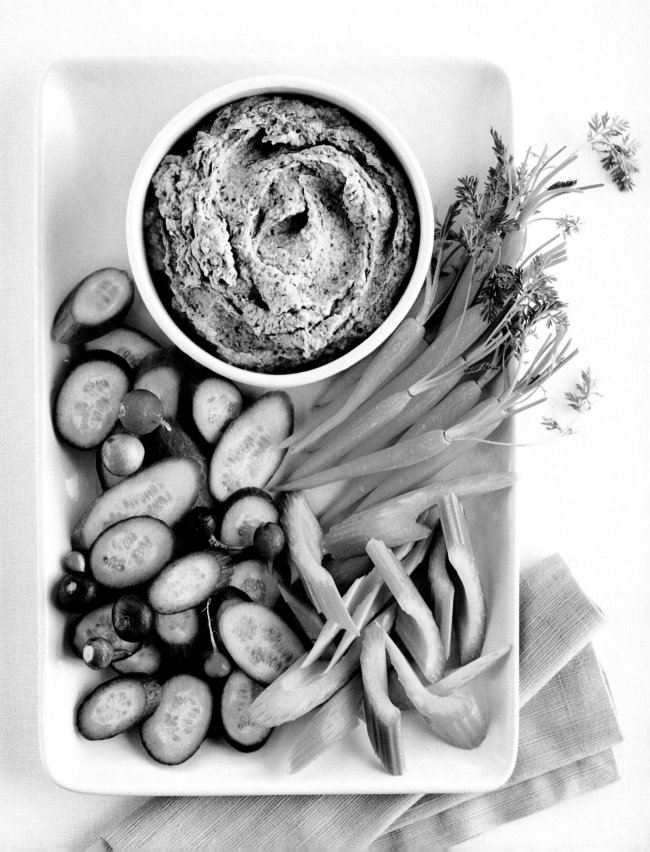

Easy Microwave Eggplant Dip for Crudités

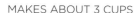

MAKES ABOUT 3 CUPS

1 large eggplant (1 to 1¼ pounds)

1 15-ounce can no-salt-added white beans, rinsed and drained

3 tablespoons fresh lemon juice

3 tablespoons tahini (sesame paste)

1 garlic clove

Salt and pepper

1. Pierce the eggplant all over with a fork. Place on a paper-towel-lined microwave-safe plate. Microwave on high for 5 minutes, turn over, and microwave until the skin collapses and the flesh is very tender, about 5 minutes longer. Let cool.

2. Remove and discard the stem, then cut in half lengthwise. Scoop out the flesh with a spoon and transfer to a food processor; discard the peel. Add the beans, lemon juice, tahini, and garlic. Process until smooth and creamy. (If you don't have a food processor, combine the eggplant, beans, lemon juice, and tahini in a bowl. Finely chop the garlic, add it to the mixture, and mash everything together. It will be a bit chunky.)

3. Season to taste with salt and pepper, cover, and refrigerate until cold. The dip can be refrigerated for up to 2 days. Serve with your favorite crudités.

Broccoli with Parmesan Crumbs

SERVES 4

Salt and freshly ground black pepper

1 pound broccoli florets

1 slice whole-wheat bread

2 tablespoons extra-virgin olive oil

1 small shallot, finely chopped

¼ cup freshly grated Parmesan cheese

1. Bring a large, deep skillet of water to boiling. Add 1 teaspoon salt, then the broccoli. Cook until bright green and just tender, about 3 minutes. Drain well and transfer to a serving plate.

2. Meanwhile, pulse the bread in a food processor to form coarse crumbs.

3. Heat the oil in the same skillet over medium-high heat. Add the shallot and cook until just browned and tender, about 2 minutes. Add the bread crumbs and cook, stirring, until evenly golden brown and crisp, about 4 minutes. Remove from the heat and stir in the cheese and a pinch of pepper.

4. Spoon the crumbs over the broccoli.

La Leche League Baking Mix

MAKES ABOUT 11 CUPS

8 cups whole-wheat flour

1 cup dry milk powder

5 tablespoons baking powder

1 tablespoon salt

1½ cups canola oil

1. Combine the flour, milk powder, baking powder, and salt in a very large bowl.

2. Add the oil and stir into the dry ingredients until the mixture is crumbly and resembles coarse meal.

3. Transfer to an airtight container, seal, and refrigerate for up to 1 week.

Muffins from La Leche League Baking Mix

MAKES 1 DOZEN

¼ cup packed brown sugar

1 cup whole milk

4 tablespoons (½ stick) butter, melted and cooled

1 large egg, beaten

½ teaspoon ground cinnamon

3 cups La Leche League Baking Mix (page 97)

1 cup dried cranberries or raisins

½ cup chopped nuts or seeds, optional

1. Preheat the oven to 425°F. Line 12 muffin cups with paper liners.

2. Beat the sugar, milk, butter, egg, and cinnamon in a large bowl until well blended. Add the baking mix and stir just until evenly moistened. Fold in the dried fruit and nuts until evenly dispersed.

3. Divide the batter among the muffin cups.

4. Bake until a toothpick inserted in the center of one comes out clean, about 23 minutes. Let cool in the pan on a wire rack for 5 minutes, then cool completely on the rack.

Banana-Nut Bread

MAKES 1 LOAF

1 cup unbleached all-purpose flour

1 cup whole-wheat flour

1 teaspoon baking soda

¼ teaspoon salt

1¼ cups mashed ripe banana (about 3 bananas)

1 teaspoon pure vanilla extract

½ cup (1 stick) butter, softened

1 cup sugar

2 large eggs

½ cup chopped walnuts, optional

1. Preheat the oven to 350°F. Grease a 9-by-5-inch loaf pan.

2. Sift together the flours, baking soda, and salt into a medium bowl. Stir together the bananas and vanilla in a small bowl.

3. Combine the butter and sugar in a large bowl. Beat with an electric mixer on medium-high speed until pale and fluffy. Add the eggs, one at a time, beating well after each addition.

4. Beat in one-third of the dry ingredients on low speed until incorporated. Beat in half of the banana mixture, then another third of the dry ingredients. Repeat once more, beating until the mixture is smooth. Stir in the nuts.

5. Transfer the batter to the prepared loaf pan. Bake until a toothpick inserted in the center comes out clean, about 1 hour 10 minutes.

6. Let cool in the pan on a wire rack for 5 minutes. Invert out of the pan and let cool completely on the wire rack.

Oatmeal Raisin Cookies

MAKES ABOUT 4 DOZEN

1 cup all-purpose flour

1 cup whole-wheat flour

1 teaspoon baking powder

1 teaspoon baking soda

1 teaspoon salt

1 cup (2 sticks) butter, softened

1 cup granulated sugar

1 cup brown sugar

2 large eggs

2 tablespoons whole milk

2 teaspoons pure vanilla extract

2½ cups old-fashioned (rolled) oats

2 cups raisins

1 cup chopped pecans or walnuts, optional

1. Preheat the oven to 350°F. Line 2 large baking sheets with parchment paper.

2. Whisk together the flours, baking powder, baking soda, and salt in a medium bowl.

3. Combine the butter and sugars in a large bowl. Beat with an electric mixer on medium-high speed until the mixture is pale and fluffy. Add the eggs, one at a time, beating well after each addition. Beat in the milk, then the vanilla.

4. Beat in the flour mixture on low speed until just incorporated. Use a wooden spoon to stir in the oats, raisins, and nuts.

5. Form the dough into 1-inch balls and place them on the prepared sheets, spacing them 1½ inches apart.

6. Bake until golden brown around the edges but pale golden in the centers, 13 to 15 minutes, rotating the baking sheets halfway through.

7. Let cool on the sheets on a wire rack for 2 minutes. Transfer to the wire rack to cool completely.

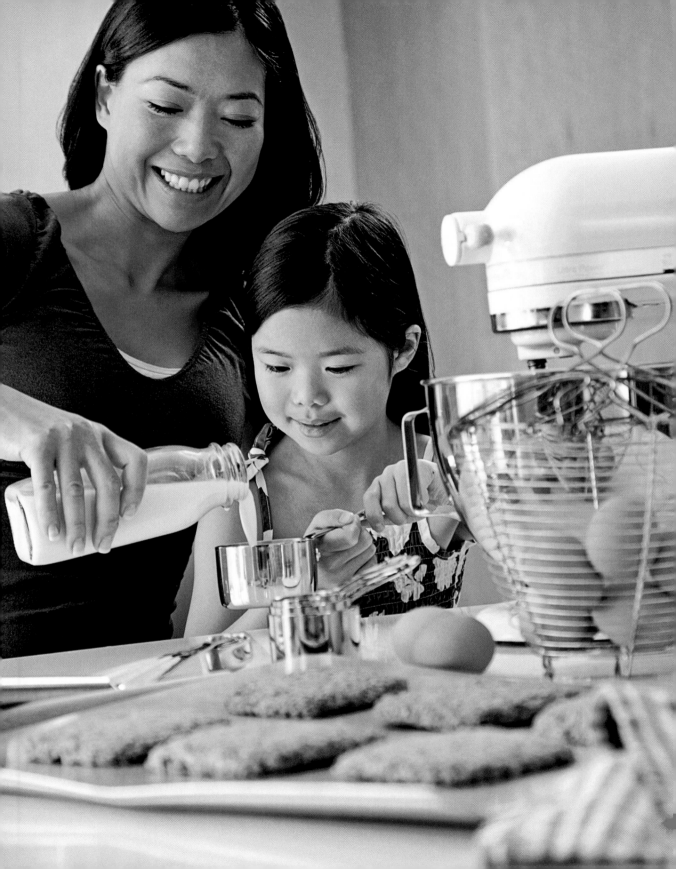

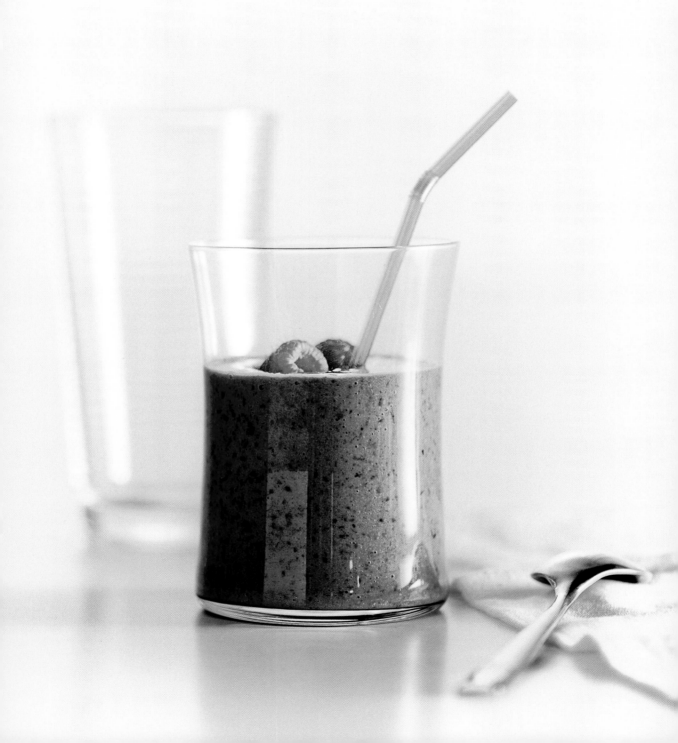

Super Smoothie with Yogurt, Berries, and Bananas

MAKES 1 SMOOTHIE

1 cup frozen berries (strawberries, blueberries, raspberries, or a combination)

1 very ripe banana

1 cup plain low-fat yogurt

½ cup pomegranate juice

1 tablespoon sugar, or to taste

1. Combine all of the ingredients in a blender. Puree until smooth, scraping down the sides of the blender as needed.

2. Taste and add more sugar if desired.

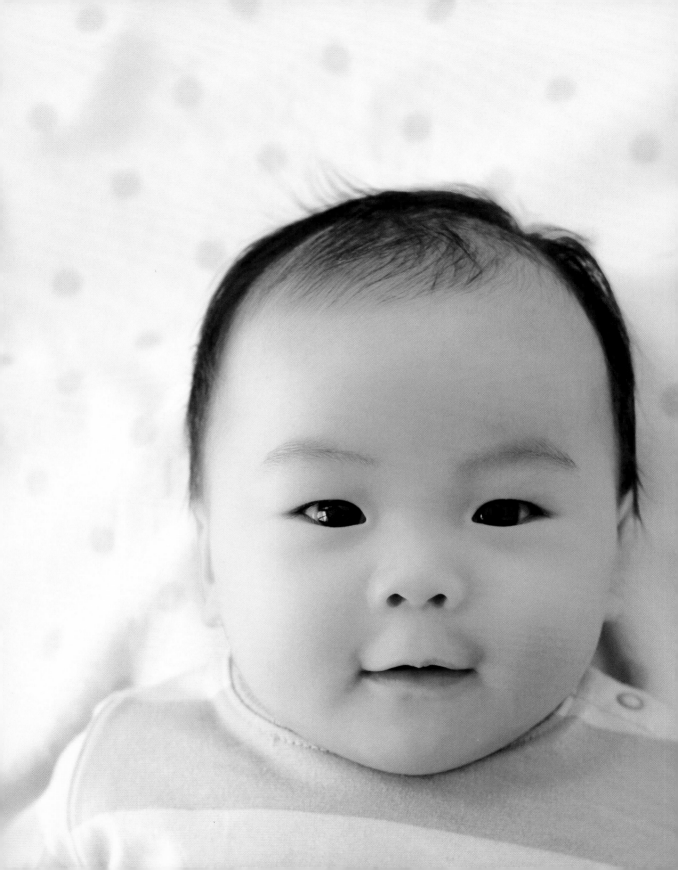

Chapter 3

Nourishing Yourself, Nourishing Your Family

FROM 6 WEEKS TO 6 MONTHS

We like to think of this postnewborn phase as "hitting your stride," when breastfeeding has become thoroughly integrated with your lifestyle. By six weeks, you and your nursling have emerged from the newborn cocoon, and you're feeling increasingly confident about breastfeeding **and** balancing the demands of the world around you. That's not to say this motherhood phase is a walk in the park (even a walk in the park with a darling baby has its challenges), but as you watch your new child grow and thrive, things feel just a little more manageable with each passing day.

We acknowledge that there is a huge difference between a 6-week-old infant and a 6-month-old baby. However, even by 6 weeks breastfeeding has become an integral part of your lives, and you know a lot more now than you did when you first held this little person. By 4 months, you're easily reading her facial cues—such as the smile that says, "Hi, Mom!" or the frown that's telling you, "But I wasn't finished nursing yet!" She's vocalizing more, too, and truly communicating, making it easier for you to figure out what she wants, when she wants it. Your relationship is increasingly interactive as your baby tunes in to you and her stimulating environment. This is an exciting time—one of many that await you—as you get increasing glimpses of your child's personality!

During this period, you'll notice that some of your routines from before you had a child are starting to come back into focus. Because your baby's eating and sleeping patterns are easier to anticipate as the weeks turn to months, your own eating and sleeping routine is becoming more consistent. Depending on your baby's age and how well you recovered from childbirth, you may be ready to do things such as exercise with more regularity. If you're taking care of yourself, resting, and eating properly, with each day you feel physically stronger and capable of doing just a bit more. If you're on maternity leave and going back to work soon, the logistics of returning to your job—from continuing with nursing to securing quality child care to fitting back into your prepregnancy clothes—are an important concern.

A normal, sit-down breakfast, lunch, and dinner are becoming daily possibilities . . . and realities. You're still doing mini-meals and snacks while you breastfeed on demand, but today you had time to make pancakes for everyone. Tomorrow you may get your favorite dinner cooking. This weekend is your older child's fourth birthday and you may even bake cupcakes—but if her grandma offers to bake them, don't say no!

Speaking of offers of help, the "Can I bring you a meal?" ones may not be coming so fast and furious now that your newborn is no longer new. Though you can continue to tap into your support network for other things, it's changing and growing as your baby does—becoming less a newborn resource and more an established mother-to-mother community as you and your child head out into the world together.

At this stage, you've mastered the art of nourishing your nursling . . . but don't forget that you still need to nourish yourself with good food. But before we consider what's best to eat right now, let's answer the question of **how** you eat.

And Baby Makes Three: Adjusting to the New Dinner Hour

If this is your first child, you may be thinking a lot about how things used to be when it was just you and your partner, compared with how different your life is

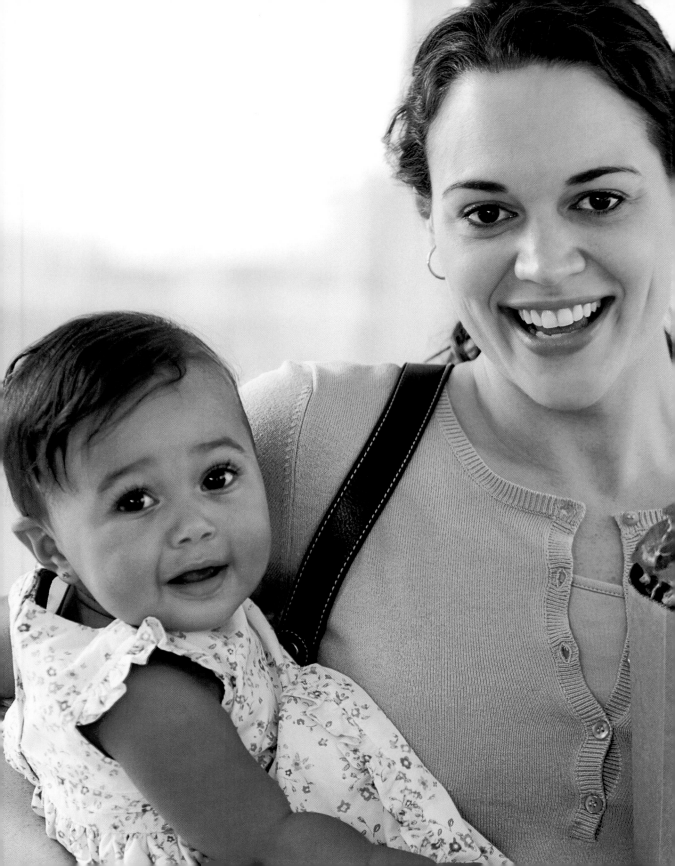

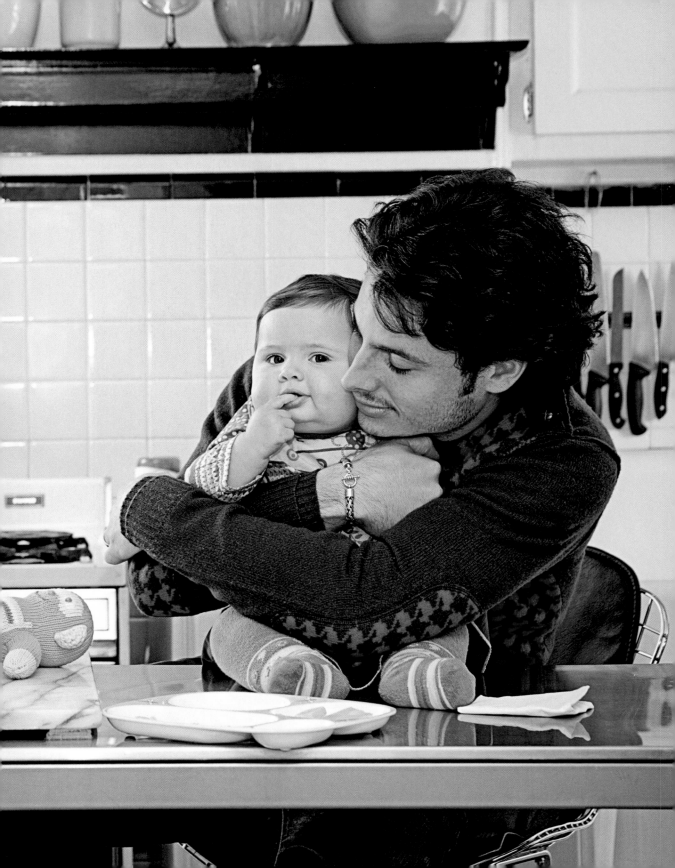

now. For many busy childless couples, a lot of quality and leisure time revolves around preparing meals and sharing them at the dinner table, or heading to a favorite restaurant, perhaps with friends.

Now that your household includes a little one, going to that restaurant may be more complicated. You can no longer decide what you want for dinner at the eleventh hour and not worry about what time you'll eat, whether a recipe is particularly complicated or time-consuming, or if it means a trip to the grocery store. Perhaps your old Saturday night routine involved dinner out followed by a movie, or cooking up a multicourse feast together at home on your own time. Babies, particularly first ones, are powerful shapers of our daily rhythms, including when, where, and how we eat!

In the early weeks, you don't miss those old routines so much. Who has the energy for an 8:00 p.m. dinner reservation, anyway, or the desire to spend precious free time on your feet and in the kitchen chopping parsley? After a while, however, particularly if you enjoy food and cooking, you may start to feel the pull back to the table for a "real meal," or the urge to return to the kitchen to whip up your Friday night favorites. This is especially true if making and sharing food is part of the way you and your partner connect after a busy day apart.

If you're ready to ease back into the kitchen and fill your house with the aromas of the home-cooked food you've been craving, here are some tips for making it easier.

Time it right. Only you know when you have those windows of free time during your nursling's naps or quiet times. Don't start a time-consuming cooking task too close to a feeding or just as he's waking and wants to be with you. Give yourself plenty of prep time—a recipe that used to take you a half hour from start to finish can require triple the time if you're stopping to nurse or take care of her other needs. Many couples like to eat an evening meal together after the baby is down for the night (even if he'll be up in few hours), but you probably want dinner, not a midnight snack.

Let your partner help. That should be your mantra by now, and not just when it comes to mealtime! Don't worry if the carrots aren't perfectly diced into uniform cubes—this is real life, not a cooking show. And make sure you have a cooking and cleaning agreement—that is, if you do the cooking, your partner cleans up the kitchen and washes the dishes.

Don't overdo it. Now is not the time to make the turkey and trimmings for Thanksgiving. If you enjoy cooking and eating, just start with whatever appeals, but keep it simple. No individual soufflés for eight guests, please. Being challenged in the kitchen can be fun—when you have time, energy, and a table waiting at that little bistro if it doesn't work out. But it's still a little early to do a Julia Child star turn. (A reminder: the original easy-to-prepare recipes throughout this book are designed for moms just like you!)

Keep baby nearby, safely. If your baby is content to rest in an infant carrier, bouncy seat (on the floor, not the table), or swing while you chop and sauté, it's the safest place for her. Don't wear your baby while you are cooking at a hot stove, opening the oven, using knives or other sharp equipment, or handling something hot that could spill or splatter. (Some moms wear their nurslings safely in a backpack-style carrier to do some kitchen chores, but generally back carriers are designed for older babies, ages 5–6 months and up.)

Play to your audience. For many a nursling, being alert in the kitchen while Mom cooks is an exciting sensory experience—the light and colors, the aromas of the family kitchen, the flash of shiny pots and pans, the sound of a loving voice (talk to your baby while you work), and watching Mommy cross from one side of this interesting room to the other. Baby can't wait to help!

"Dinner times are crunch times—there's no doubt. Some things we've found helpful: In the colder months we make soup on the weekends (it keeps for several days and works well for an easy reheat). The slow cooker is making a well-deserved comeback. And we make more than enough chicken (for example) for a meal one day, then dice it up and make chicken enchiladas the next, or a salad, etc. I try to slice and dice enough veggies for several meals at one time to keep in the fridge."

And Baby Makes Four (or Five or . . .): The New Family Meal

If you have an older child or children, you face a different set of mealtime challenges than you did with your singleton, particularly if big sister or brother is still a little one. Older kids can be very helpful in and out of the kitchen, but toddlers and preschoolers are barely out of babyhood themselves and have a way of demanding your attention just when you are heating up the olive oil. (They seem drawn like magnets to that hot spot right between you and the stove!) Here are some mom-tested ideas that have worked for mothers of two, three, four, and counting. . . .

Make a game out of work. Give big brother or sister age-appropriate chores such as setting the table, folding napkins, rinsing dishes, or cleaning the counters. (Water-filled spray bottles make this last one fun, though be prepared for errant squirts!) For little kids, doing a grown-up job is more of a treat than a task.

"Read me a story, Mommy." You can't right this minute, but someone else can—keep a CD or MP3 player in the kitchen so your kids can listen to their favorite recorded stories and follow along with the book (great for pre-readers and brand-new ones). If you have a computer in the kitchen, keep it "tuned" to interactive, educational games and websites.

Connect the dots. Go low-tech and keep a stash of activity books, pencils, and markers handy. Books of mazes, color-by-numbers, and connect-the-dots are classic ways to pass the time at the kitchen table. Some kids go for educational activities such as math puzzles or word games—but keep it fun and not frustrating, since you can't focus on helping right now.

Craft and cook. Children who like crafts or art projects will keep themselves busy, but experienced moms know that dinnertime is not the time for messy paint and lots of glitter! Again, keep it simple and fun; when you're trying to get a meal cooked, you don't have time (or the extra hands) to help glue the googly eyes on just so.

Have a sing-along. While you cook and baby is safe on the floor, have a sing-along and let your older child play an instrument as she entertains her sibling, even if it's just banging out a rhythm with a pot and spoon.

Let them play with their food. Your older child may want to do what you're doing—cooking! Stirring, pouring, mixing, and measuring are just some things kids can do in the kitchen. Depending on their age and skills, big kids may be able to operate small mini-choppers (with enclosed blades) under your supervision, to cut up items such as vegetables and herbs. Little ones can "work" at the kitchen counter or table next to Mom, with their own stash of dough (real or play), a rolling pin, and cookie cutters.

Big girls (and boys) do cry. And siblings often do it just as things are really heating up in the kitchen. **He took my bear. . . . She pushed me. . . . Mommy!** "Figure out who needs what the most," a mother of three says. "You get good at this! Remind the older ones, 'I get worried when you scream like that.' They will get the message." And older kids sometimes get very good at being responsible for younger family members—thank them for being good caregivers and helpers!

Send them packing. Well, not exactly, but school-age kids who aren't making themselves useful in the kitchen usually have homework that should begin before dinnertime. A simple "Don't you have something to do for school?" will send them scurrying for their backpacks. And if it's nice outside and they're homework free, "Why don't you play outside?" works too.

Silence the growling. Tummies, that is. Older kids often darken the door of the kitchen during dinner prep because they're absolutely starving. Make sure to keep healthy snacks on hand, including fresh fruit, cut-up veggies, low-fat yogurt, nuts, whole-grain pretzels and crackers, homemade trail mix, and so on. (The same healthy snacks you should have on hand for yourself are often perfect for your kids.)

Invite them in. Children who help prepare the family meal generally eat more healthfully and are more willing to try new foods (that they helped make) than kids who rarely venture into the kitchen. Depending on

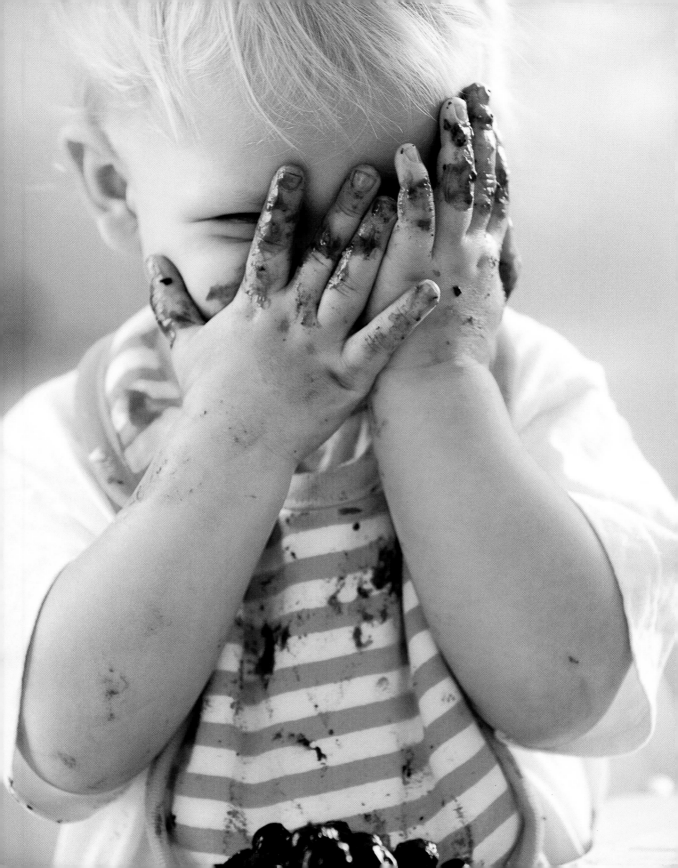

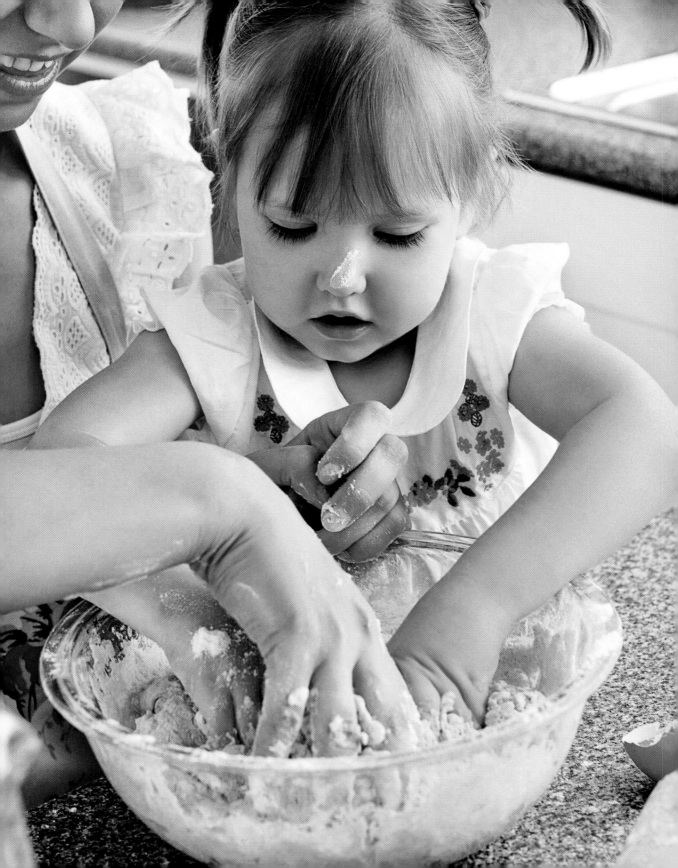

their ages, let your kids help make and serve food. They may be more capable than you think. (If you are a working mother with younger kids who need supervision, "kids in the kitchen" often works best on weekends and not weeknights when you're feeling rushed.)

Partner with your partner. All of the suggestions above put you, Mom, on the front lines of food prep, but don't go it alone, especially in the evenings. If your spouse or partner enjoys cooking, by all means back away from the stove! If they aren't keen on the kitchen, their parenting skills—nuzzling your nursling, playing or helping with older kids—are in demand.

Food, Glorious Food!

This idea—which takes potluck to a whole new level and saves you time and work—came from Inbal Bahar, an LLLI volunteer, doula, and mother of three:

> During the December holiday season, I noticed that we potlucked a lot, or just went over to friends' for meals. Suddenly I noticed that we weren't cooking as much, but still eating well. I was thinking about it one night while lying in bed. And then it hit me. Exchanging food with friends on a regular basis is the answer to spending less time cooking but still eating a healthy diet! I shared this idea with two friends, who have children close in age to ours, and they were very enthusiastic.
>
> We worked it out so that each family is assigned a day of the week (Mondays, Wednesdays, or Fridays), makes a main dish on that day, and delivers it to the other two families before suppertime. So, for example, if I make a red lentil lasagna on a Monday, I triple my recipe and make three lasagnas, then deliver the food to the other two families. On Wednesdays and Fridays, the other two families do the same and bring a main dish for supper to me. I end

Food, Glorious Food! (CONTINUED)

up cooking on just one of those days, sharing the food, and getting two other wonderful suppers I didn't have to work for.

What we got out of this food exchange (or FEX) was homemade, nutritious, and diverse "adult" food (available for the children, too). I find that this FEX arrangement works best for families who are at a similar stage in life and like-minded in their food philosophy. To make sure our FEX works smoothly, we email each other on "our" day and let the others know what we are making and if we advise them to prepare a salad or a grain to go with the main dish.

I think our FEX is a simple and elegant idea for families who like to eat home-cooked meals without spending a lot of time making them. It only works, however, if all the families are committed, reliable, and really enjoy this arrangement. FEX made my life easier. Maybe it can make yours easier, too! Give it a try.[1]

Reduce the stress and increase the pleasures of dinner (and other meals) by "FEX"-ing it, and look for recipes in these pages that are freezer-friendly, make-ahead, or quick (active prep time 30 minutes or less)—see the lists on pages 79–80, 217–18, and 116–17. As you ease back into the kitchen and plan meals, remember the blueprint for healthy eating (page 8)—lean protein, complex carbohydrates, plenty of vegetables and fruit (and dairy, if you eat it). One more component of a healthy meal? Enjoyment! **Bon appétit!**

⚡ Quick Recipes: Active Prep Time Under 30 Minutes

- Bacon and Spinach Pasta, page 45
- Baked Salmon with Apricot Glaze, page 178
- Black Bean Salsa, page 144
- Broccoli Pesto Multigrain Pasta, page 179

- Broccoli with Parmesan Crumbs, page 96
- Celery Root and Potato Puree, page 187
- Chicken and Sugar Snap Pea Sauté, page 88
- Chicken Tomato Quesadillas, page 223
- Corn Bread (page 145), Muffins (page 98), Pancakes (page 234), and Waffles (page 233) from La Leche League Baking Mix
- Crab Tostadas, page 91
- Hummus, page 183
- Orange-Braised Baby Carrots, page 186
- Oven-Baked Chicken Tenders, page 222
- Prune-Stuffed Pork Tenderloin, page 132
- Roasted Brussels Sprouts, page 140
- Roasted Mushrooms with Shallots and Parsley, page 142
- Roasted Salmon with Light Horseradish Sour Cream Sauce, page 35
- Sautéed Spinach with Garlic, page 51
- Soft Scrambled Eggs with Leeks, page 181
- Soy-Lime Marinated Salmon, page 133
- Summer Squash Omelets, page 180
- Super Smoothie with Yogurt, Berries, and Bananas, page 103
- Three Bears Porridge, page 147
- UFOs (Unidentified Frying Objects), page 232
- Whole-Wheat Spaghetti with Anchovies and Cauliflower, page 90

From Waiting for Baby to Baby Weight

Breastfeeding is important in many ways that you may already be aware of, from the innumerable lasting health benefits that it offers your baby to the wide-ranging ways that breastfeeding maximizes your own health—including a jump-start on postpartum weight loss, protection against breast, uterine, and cervical cancers, and so much more. It's often the weight loss, however, that emerges as one of the first noticeable benefits.

Breastfeeding naturally causes the uterus to contract thanks to the release of the hormone oxytocin, which helps to shrink the belly back to a size resembling its prepregnancy state. (Oxytocin can do only so much, however—if you want abs of steel, you'll have to put in some additional work later!) Breastfeeding also uses up calories, as much as 500 a day depending on various factors.

There is a relationship between how much weight you gained during pregnancy and how much weight you retain postpartum; if you gained more than what was necessary (based on your BMI), it follows that you'll have more to get rid of, and furthermore, your body will try to hang on to the extra fat. This is Mother Nature at work, because the hormones that assist in milk production also support the retention of fat. Your fat stores provide about 100 calories daily of energy for you to produce milk, so your body is reluctant to throw off this security blanket. Mother Nature isn't trying to goad you into redefining fat stores as the place where you have to shop for jeans; she's simply supporting your efforts to nourish your hungry baby.

"Give yourself some time to heal and get used to breastfeeding and motherhood before you worry about the weight. No one except you is noticing it . . . they are all looking at the baby, not you."

However, over time—unless you take in more calories than your body needs—you should experience weight loss during breastfeeding. It may not come as rapidly as your best friend's, or it may be faster than your sister-in-law's. As you're already discovering, mothers have many things in common, but our differences are equally notable.

What to Eat Now

To stay healthy and maintain consistent breastfeeding, you should continue to strive for the recommended levels of protein, calcium, iron, folate, fiber, and other nutrients such as magnesium, potassium, and zinc that we discussed in previous chapters. (Refer to pages 61–62 for recommended postpartum nutrient levels and pages 10–11, 12–14, and 72–73 for food sources).

If you are aiming to return to your prepregnancy weight or to reach a healthy BMI through dieting, eating nutritiously is a must—and doing so is much easier if you keep the right foods in your house. When you choose nutrient-dense meals or snacks that fill you up (the turkey wrap instead of the instant mac and cheese, the juicy apple or handful of almonds instead of the potato chips), you naturally make better calorie choices.

During the first 6 months of breastfeeding, many nursing mothers lose about 1¾ pounds per month. (To lose 1 pound, you must expend 3,500 calories more than you consume.) Aim for no more than 1 pound a week. Crash diets, trendy weight-loss programs, or other plans that promise fast shedding of pounds are not recommended because they may interfere with the essential vitamins and nutrients that you need right now to stay healthy and energetic for yourself and your baby. In addition, environmental pollutants, such as PCBs and pesticides, are naturally stored in your body fat. If you lose weight too rapidly, these contaminants can enter your milk supply.

Many diet and lactation experts suggest that nursing mothers consume a minimum of 1,500 to 1,800 calories per day to maintain their milk supply; check with your doctor before you start a weight loss program or significantly reduce your calorie intake. It is possible to lose weight safely through diet and exercise during breastfeeding.

Exercise: The Way to Really Tip the Scales (in the Right Direction)

You already know that breastfeeding on its own burns hundreds of calories a day, but if you really want to safely nudge your postpartum weight loss along, adding regular exercise to your daily routine will burn additional calories and help you regain your muscle tone. Studies have shown that mothers lose fat from their hips and thighs more easily during breastfeeding than at other times; in addition, weight loss among nursing mothers is greatest 3 to 6 months postpartum. Take advantage of this potential weight loss window by adding daily exercise to your healthy eating habits.

If you're an avid exerciser, you probably have already gotten out there to run,

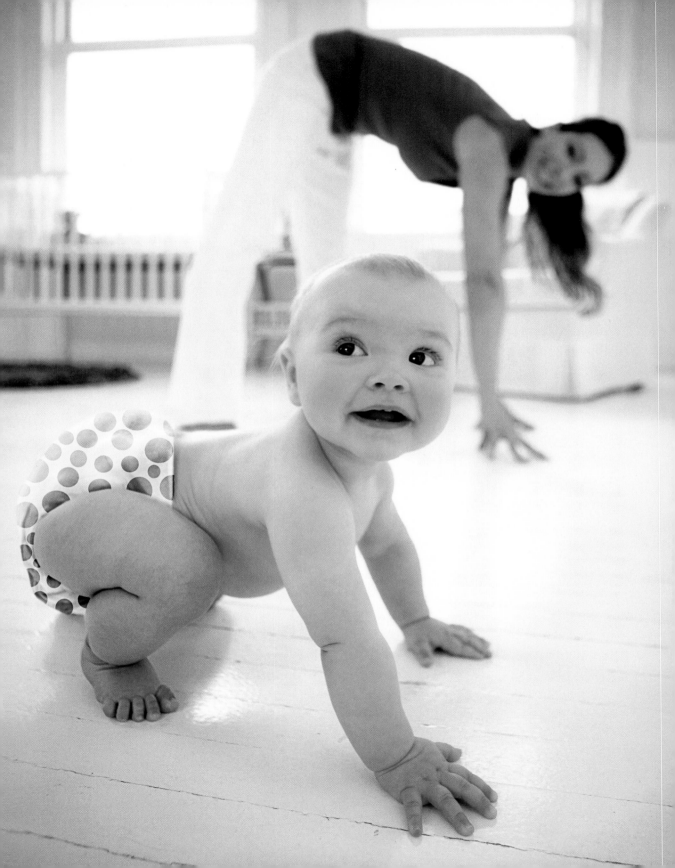

bike, swim, or do the Downward Dog. But if you have yet to move it, shake it, or stretch it out, just start with walking with your baby for a half hour a day and work up from there. If you wear your nursling in a sling or other carrier, that's even better; weight-bearing exercise is an excellent way to strength-train, and your growing baby definitely counts! Find a group of like-minded moms and walk together with your little ones. Look for mom-and-baby exercise classes in your community; many popular "boot camp" classes designed for mothers are baby-friendly. If you can't get outside because of the weather, dance with your baby (or dance by yourself when he's napping), or find an indoor workout routine that you like.

Normal exercise will not impact the quality or quantity of your milk production, though you should wear a good, supportive bra; nurse before you work out so that your breasts are less full; and your nursling might appreciate it if you take a quick shower before her next meal! Exercise will benefit both of you, so however you do it and whatever you do, as they say: just do it.

Eating Right, Feeling Good: LLLI Moms Share Their Ideas

"Some good healthy 'convenience' foods: premixed salad, baby carrots, broccoli florets, corn tortillas (sprinkle on a little cheese and nuke or toast in toaster oven), apples—whole or cut up—brown rice (premade, you just have to reheat), cereal with milk, yogurt, cottage cheese, frozen fruit."

"Peanut butter or sunflower butter [a spreadable, peanut-free alternative made from sunflower seeds]! Just stick to the proper serving size. PB is great on rice crisps, carrots, celery, or a slice of bread. . . . Light yogurt is amazing with almonds, granola, or fresh berries mixed in. I like to eat it as dessert. It's frozen-yogurty if you stick it in the freezer a couple of hours prior to eating. . . . Buy fruit and veggies, cut them up in advance, and store them in a jar. This way, when hunger strikes, your healthy snack is ready for you. It'll

---

Eating Right, Feeling Good: LLLI Moms Share Their Ideas

(CONTINUED)

protect you from eating things that'll pack on the pounds. . . . I get really hungry while I'm away from home, so I store granola bars in my car and purse. It saves me a lot of money and I don't opt for candy bars at the gas station this way! . . . Water! Carry a water bottle with you when you leave home. Drink it when you start feeling a bit hungry and it'll help you to eat a little less. . . . In an ideal world, one would follow the food pyramid as closely as possible. It's important to make sure you eat lots of healthy fruits and vegetables (avoid juice when you can, as it's a very high-sugar substitute for fruits/veggies). Also find out what the right amount of protein is for your height/weight, and eat just that (not more than the suggested amount because many proteins are also high in fat and calories)."

"Just walking regularly and nursing and eating healthy—you will be surprised how much weight you do lose without dieting."

Places to Go, People to See: Eating Well When You're on the Move

Now that you are becoming more mobile with your nursling, taking walks, meeting friends, running errands, or maybe even getting on a plane or going on a road trip to visit the new grandparents, you've discovered firsthand just how convenient breastfeeding is. You don't need to carry along bottles or any other items to feed your baby. You've got everything you need 24/7—for baby, that is.

Don't Forget Your Food

Make room in the diaper bag for your own stash of healthy snacks and portable meals (don't forget the utensils and napkins). The ideas in Chapters 1 and 2, as well as the suggestions from LLLI moms we've been sharing in this chapter, should get you started.

Try to avoid getting caught without food when you're on the go, so that you don't find yourself at a convenience store or at an airport newsstand or fast-food outlet, trying to find an unprocessed, low-fat, low-sugar snack or meal that will give you energy. Read the labels before you settle for that "healthful" granola bar—you may be better off with a dark chocolate bar studded with almonds, and some milk. And stay hydrated—put that cup holder on the back of the stroller to good use!

Working Moms Get Hungry, Too

If you are returning to work now, one major change you'll notice right away is that your three-meals-a-day schedule gets back on track (assuming your job spans a regular 9-to-5 time frame) fast, out of necessity. To keep your energy up, don't skip breakfast, bring along a midmorning snack, don't wait too long for lunch, and eat something in the late afternoon between lunch and dinner. When you pack up your pumping supplies (it helps to do this the night before), organize your food, too. Prepare or pack up as much as you can when you're not rushed. You may have a good take-out place or market near your workplace, but generally, food you bring from home is going to be the best bet nutritionally (and you'll save money, too).

Many working mothers who express milk during lunchtime get really good at pumping, talking on the phone, or working at the computer, and eating lunch, all at the same time! It's not the ideal scenario, of course (and it depends largely on the conditions under which you pump at work), but you'll get into a groove soon enough that works for you.

If you're fortunate enough to have on-site child care or your baby's caregiver is close enough so that you can breastfeed during the day, take food, snacks,

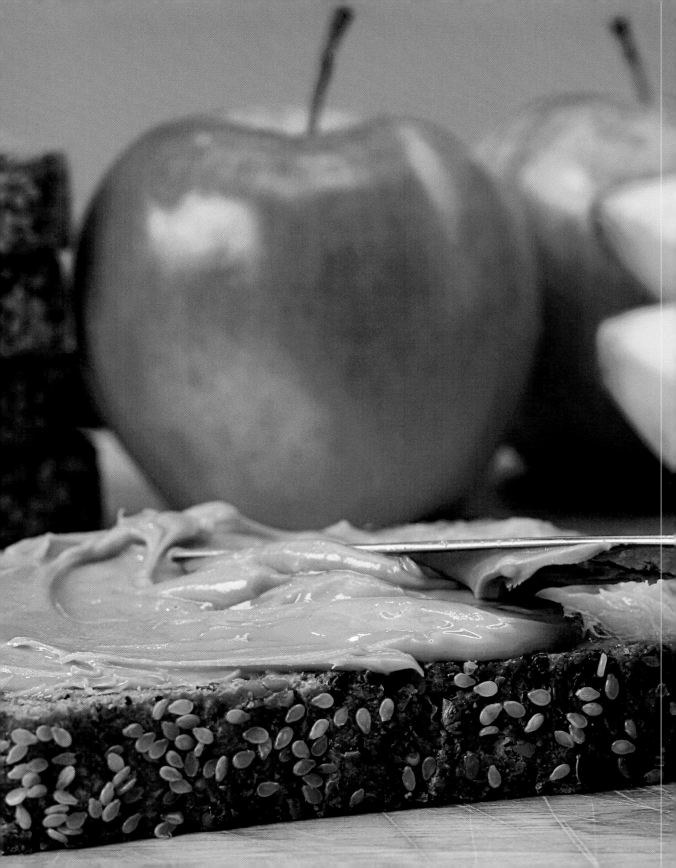

and drinks with you when you are nursing. Balancing work and nursing is demanding, so staying healthy through eating well is especially important. You do have to do more advance planning, but ultimately, whether you're at work or at home, on the road or nesting in your living room, the rule remains the same: eat to hunger, drink to thirst.

Can I Eat This?

By now, you probably have figured out what foods might cause your nursling to have a little (or a lot) of extra gas, or why you need to rethink that iced coffee. As you continue your return to prepregnancy eating habits and patterns (the healthy ones only, we hope), you are probably reintroducing some "old" foods into your diet. Most of the foods that you were advised to skip during pregnancy, such as certain soft cheeses, are perfectly safe to eat now.

Check with your doctor if you're not sure, but if you are healthy, there is almost nothing you can't eat during breastfeeding. If you consume the following items, note these precautions:

"I ate while pumping for many months . . . but I did save a lot of money, taking my lunch to work every day, and got into a good habit with that."

"Both my breaks and my lunch will be spent pumping. I only get 30 minutes for lunch. But I know this doesn't last forever, so I can do it if needed."

Some herbs. Sage, peppermint, and parsley, when consumed in large amounts, are linked to lowered volumes of milk production. In fact, these culinary herbs are sometimes recommended if there is a reason for abrupt weaning or for controlling an oversupply of breast milk.

There are also several medicinal herbs, such as rhubarb root, aloe, and maté, that are contraindicated during lactation. **Medications and Mothers' Milk** by Thomas Hale is a resource used by pharmacists, lactation consultants, and other professionals; it contains updated listings of contraindicated herbs for nursing mothers. Most culinary herbs, especially in the quantities generally called for in typical recipes, are completely safe to eat; if you're not sure, find out.

Sushi. Federal regulations require that fish that will be eaten raw (with the exception of tuna) must be frozen in order to kill parasites and certain bacteria. (Though this is a federal requirement, it's up to local health officials to enforce it.) Properly handled fish for sushi should not be a problem—the problem is whether you can know for sure that it's been properly handled. Buy your sushi from a trusted source; be careful with prepackaged supermarket sushi unless you know for sure that it's been freshly made and safely refrigerated.

Mercury remains a concern postpartum. (See page 32 for information on the dangers of methylmercury and on the safe consumption of seafood.) Sushi-grade tuna, such as some bluefin, can be quite high in mercury. Many health professionals recommend that nursing mothers limit their sushi eating to once a week. If you're a sushi fan, ask your doctor about the latest guidelines concerning lactation and safe consumption of sushi and other seafood. Fish (cooked or raw), as mentioned before, is still a superior source of DHA, which your baby needs.

And remember, if you do eat something that disagrees with you, it's unlikely your baby will have the same reaction. You do not need to interrupt breastfeeding if you have a stomach bug that is running its normal course (there are **very** few illnesses that would require you to stop nursing, including food poisoning). Because your baby shares your immune system, you're passing along valuable antibodies during illness. If you have a stomach virus that causes vomiting and/or diarrhea, there is a chance your milk production will temporarily dip; add extra fluids to stay hydrated and your milk supply will return to normal as you recover.

Food Sensitivities and Allergies

Once your baby is about 1 month of age, he has gotten quite used to your diet through his. However, if you are starting to notice some physical reactions that seem out of the ordinary as you broaden your own diet and return to your pre-pregnancy eating patterns, they might be triggered by a food sensitivity or allergy. Some symptoms related to food allergy occur very soon after your infant has ingested the potential allergen through breast milk. These include:

- Projectile vomiting (not drooling or ordinary spit-up)
- Diarrhea
- Rash, eczema (atopic dermatitis), hives

It is very difficult to determine if a young baby has a true food allergy, but food allergies do have a genetic component. If you or your baby's father has a history of food allergies, there is an increased chance that your child will have them, too. Most food allergy reactions occur immediately.

Food allergies are exceedingly serious and can be life-threatening; however, some studies have concluded that many food allergies may be misdiagnosed and are actually food intolerances, also known as sensitivities. About 33 percent of the U.S. population believes they have food allergies; by contrast, a 2010 study commissioned by the U.S. government suggests that about 8 percent of children and fewer than 5 percent of adults have true food allergies.[2] (It should be noted that even a seemingly telltale symptom, such as eczema, may not indicate a food allergy; only a third of eczema cases are food-related. The rest are due to genetic factors.)

The most common food allergens are milk, egg, and peanut proteins, all of which can pass into your breast milk after you consume them. However, there is no definite evidence to suggest that eliminating these foods from your diet during breastfeeding (or during pregnancy) will reduce the chances of your infant developing an allergy.

Other foods in your diet that may cause a reaction in your baby include eggs, soy, tree nuts, and wheat. (Your baby may also be sensitive to caffeine, as mentioned previously, and chocolate.)

If you think there may be a link between your consumption of certain foods and the onset of symptoms such as those listed above, you could try keeping a food journal to track any connections and eliminate one food at a time, for a week or two, to see if there is a change. If your baby is exhibiting symptoms indicative of food sensitivity or allergy, ask your doctor about tailoring an eating plan to determine which foods may be causing the reactions. It is best to have a pediatric allergist diagnose food allergy through both blood tests and skin tests; if a true allergy is diagnosed, a breastfeeding mother will be encouraged to eliminate the allergen from her diet.

Research shows that exclusively breastfed babies are actually protected from food allergies later on.[3] For instance, studies have shown that babies who drink formula—made from cow's milk or soy protein—have a much greater chance of developing allergies to both milk and soy.

Do not let fears of food allergies, which are not common in most infants, interfere with nursing your baby.

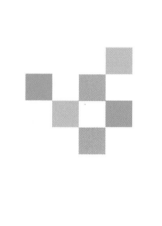

Red Onion and Olive Roasted Chicken Pieces

SERVES 4

2 tablespoons extra-virgin olive oil

2 large red onions, sliced

1 whole (3½-pound) chicken, cut into 8 pieces

2 garlic cloves, crushed

¼ teaspoon dried thyme

Salt and freshly ground black pepper

½ cup Kalamata olives, pitted and halved

1. Preheat the oven to 425°F.

2. Coat the bottom of a large rimmed baking sheet with 1 tablespoon oil. Arrange the onion slices in the pan in a single layer.

3. Toss the chicken with the garlic, thyme, and remaining oil until well coated. Arrange in a single layer on top of the onion slices and season with salt and pepper.

4. Roast for 30 minutes, then scatter the olives over the chicken. Roast until the chicken is cooked through (the juices will run clear when the chicken is pierced with the tip of a knife), about 5 minutes longer. Let the chicken rest for 5 minutes before serving.

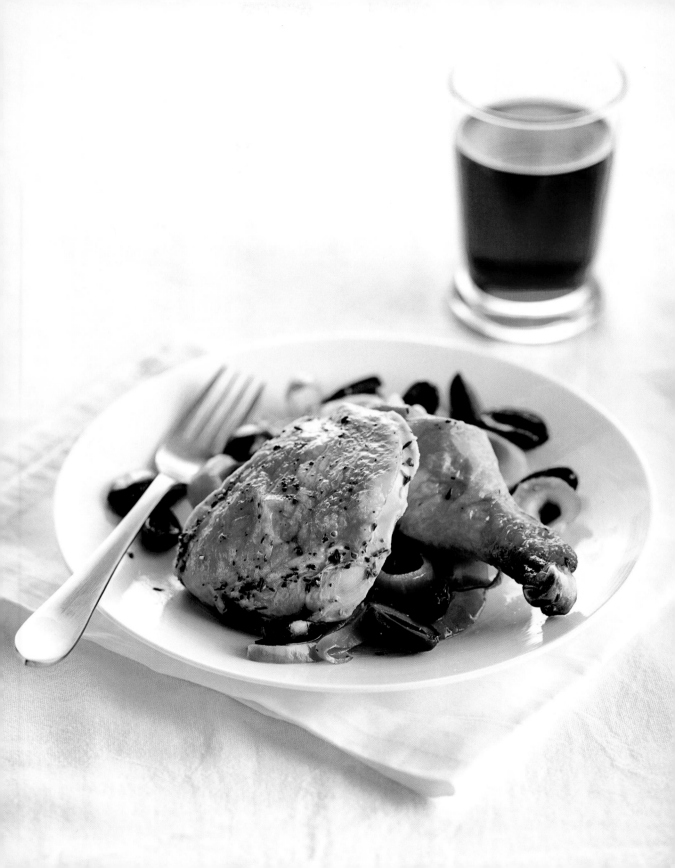

Prune-Stuffed Pork Tenderloin

SERVES 4

½ cup pitted prunes

2 tablespoons extra-virgin olive oil

1 garlic clove, minced

1½ cups thinly sliced Swiss chard leaves

Salt and freshly ground black pepper

¼ teaspoon dried thyme

1 whole (1-pound) pork tenderloin

1. Preheat the oven to 475°F. Soak the prunes in hot water.

2. Heat 1 tablespoon oil in a large ovenproof skillet over medium-high heat. Add the garlic and cook 15 seconds. Add the Swiss chard and a pinch each of salt and pepper and cook, stirring occasionally, until wilted, about 5 minutes. Stir in the thyme leaves and remove from the heat.

3. Cut a slit lengthwise along the side of the pork tenderloin, two-thirds through the thickness of the meat. Open the pork like a book. Transfer the Swiss chard mixture to the pork, spreading it in an even layer. Drain the prunes and arrange them in a line over the chard. Close the pork over the filling. Rub the outside of the pork with the remaining tablespoon oil and sprinkle with salt and pepper.

4. Wipe out the skillet and transfer the pork to the skillet, seam side down with the tapered end tucked under. Roast until the pork just loses its pinkness, about 15 minutes. Let rest for 5 minutes, then slice crosswise.

Soy-Lime Marinated Salmon

SERVES 4

3 tablespoons reduced-sodium soy sauce

1 tablespoon extra-virgin olive oil

1 tablespoon fresh lime juice, plus lime wedges for serving

1 green onion, finely chopped

1-inch piece fresh ginger, peeled and finely chopped

2 teaspoons sugar

4 6-ounce center-cut skinless salmon fillets

Freshly ground black pepper

1. Stir together the soy sauce, oil, lime juice, onion, ginger, and sugar until the sugar dissolves. Place the salmon in a large resealable plastic bag and pour the mixture over the fish. Seal the bag, place it in a dish, and refrigerate for at least 30 minutes and up to 2 hours.

2. Preheat the oven to 375°F. Line a rimmed baking sheet with foil.

3. Transfer the salmon from the marinade to the prepared sheet. Discard the marinade. Sprinkle the salmon with pepper.

4. Bake the salmon until just opaque throughout, about 12 minutes. A knife will pierce easily through the flesh. Serve with lime wedges.

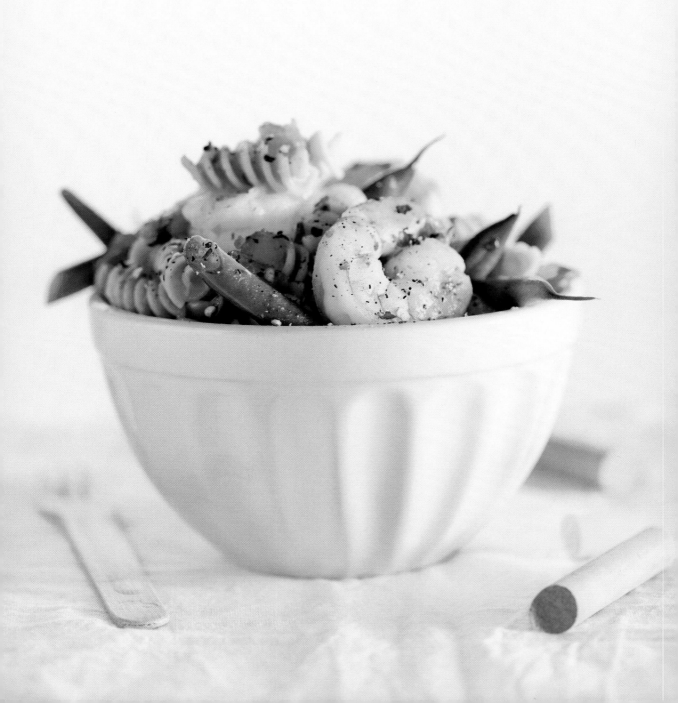

Shrimp Scampi Whole-Grain Pasta Toss

SERVES 4

1 box (13 to 14 ounces) whole-grain rotini

8 ounces green beans, trimmed and cut into 2-inch pieces

3 tablespoons extra-virgin olive oil

1 pound large shrimp, peeled and deveined

Salt and freshly ground black pepper

2 garlic cloves, finely chopped

¼ teaspoon crushed red pepper flakes, optional

1 tablespoon butter

1 tomato, cored, seeded, and chopped

1. Bring a large pot of salted water to a boil.

2. Add the pasta and cook according to the package's directions. Three minutes before the pasta is done, add the green beans. Cook with the pasta for 3 minutes. Reserve 1 cup of the pasta cooking water and drain the pasta mixture. Return the pasta to the pot.

3. Meanwhile, heat the oil in a large skillet over medium-high heat until hot. Add the shrimp in a single layer and season with salt and pepper. Cook, turning once, until just pink throughout, about 2 minutes. Use a slotted spoon to transfer the shrimp to the pot with the pasta.

4. Add the garlic to the skillet and cook, stirring, until golden, about 1 minute. Add the red pepper and cook for 15 seconds. Stir in the butter until it melts. Transfer the mixture to the pasta.

5. Add the tomato to the pasta mixture and set over medium heat. Toss until everything is well mixed, adding the reserved cooking water as needed to keep the mixture moist. Season to taste with salt and pepper.

Slow Cooker Vegetarian Chili

SERVES 4

1 15-ounce can crushed tomatoes in puree

1 cup dried black beans, soaked overnight, rinsed, and drained

5 carrots, chopped

1 large red onion, finely chopped

2 garlic cloves, finely chopped

2 tablespoons chili powder

2 teaspoons ground cumin

½ teaspoon dried oregano

Salt and freshly ground black pepper

½ cup shredded sharp cheddar cheese

¼ cup sour cream

¼ cup chopped fresh cilantro leaves

1. Combine the tomatoes and 2 cups water in a 5½-quart slow cooker.

2. Stir in the beans, carrots, onion, garlic, chili powder, cumin, oregano, and a pinch each of salt and pepper. Cover and cook on low for 8 hours or on high for 6 hours. It is done when the beans and vegetables are tender.

3. Serve with the cheese, sour cream, and cilantro.

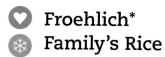

Froehlich*
Family's Rice

SERVES 8

3 bacon strips

1 medium onion, chopped

½ green bell pepper, finely chopped

2 cups brown rice

Salt and freshly ground black pepper

2 pounds ground beef chuck

2 28-ounce cans stewed tomatoes

½ teaspoon dried oregano

4 ounces cheddar cheese, shredded (1 cup)

*Edwina Froehlich is a co-founder of LLLI.

1. Place the bacon in a large, deep saucepot. Cook, turning occasionally, over medium heat until crisp and browned. Transfer to paper towels to drain. When cool, crumble.

2. Add the onion and pepper to the pan and cook, stirring occasionally, until tender, about 5 minutes. Stir in the rice, 1 quart water, and a pinch of salt. Bring the mixture to a boil, then cover, reduce the heat to low, and simmer for 30 minutes.

3. Meanwhile, heat a large skillet over medium-high heat. Add the beef and a pinch each of salt and pepper. Cook, stirring occasionally and breaking the meat into small chunks, until browned, about 8 minutes.

4. Add the meat, tomatoes, and oregano to the rice. Bring the mixture to a boil over medium-high heat, then reduce the heat to low and simmer until the rice is tender, about 45 minutes.

5. Divide among serving dishes and top with the cheese and bacon.

Savory Baked French Toast

SERVES 6

8 slices firm whole-wheat sandwich bread

6 ounces baby spinach

1 pound asparagus, trimmed and cut into 1-inch pieces

6 ounces sharp cheddar cheese, shredded (1½ cups)

2 cups reduced-fat (2%) milk

6 large eggs

Salt and freshly ground black pepper

1. Butter an 8-inch square (2-quart) baking dish.

2. Arrange 4 bread slices in the prepared dish in a single layer. Top with half of the spinach, asparagus, and cheese. Repeat the layering once.

3. Whisk together the milk, eggs, and a pinch each of salt and pepper. Slowly pour into the baking dish. Cover with plastic wrap and gently press down so that the bread absorbs the milk mixture. Refrigerate at least 1 hour and up to overnight.

4. When ready to bake, preheat the oven to 350°F.

5. Uncover the baking dish and bake until a knife inserted in the center comes out clean and the top is golden brown, about 1 hour. Let stand 10 minutes, then cut into pieces.

Quinoa Pilaf with White Beans, Feta Cheese, and Summer Vegetables

SERVES 4

3 cups low-sodium vegetable broth

2 cups quinoa, rinsed and drained

3 tablespoons olive oil

1 red bell pepper, stemmed, seeded, and diced

1 orange bell pepper, stemmed, seeded, and diced

2 green onions, finely chopped

1 zucchini, trimmed and diced

1 yellow summer squash, trimmed and diced

¼ teaspoon dried oregano

Salt and freshly ground black pepper

2 large tomatoes, cored, seeded, and diced

1 15-ounce can white kidney beans (cannellini), rinsed and drained

½ cup crumbled pasteurized feta cheese

3 tablespoons fresh lemon juice

2 tablespoons red wine vinegar

1. Bring the broth to a boil in a large saucepan. Stir in the quinoa. Cover, reduce the heat to low, and simmer until the quinoa is tender and the broth is absorbed, about 15 minutes. Remove from the heat and fluff with a fork.

2. Meanwhile, heat 2 tablespoons oil in a large skillet over medium-high heat. Add the peppers and half of the green onions. Cook, stirring occasionally, until just tender, about 5 minutes. Add the zucchini, yellow squash, oregano, and a pinch each of salt and pepper. Cook, stirring occasionally, until the squash is just tender, about 5 minutes.

3. Transfer the quinoa and vegetables to a large bowl. Add the tomatoes, beans, feta, lemon juice, vinegar, remaining green onions, and remaining oil. Toss until well mixed. Season to taste with salt and pepper. The pilaf can be refrigerated in an airtight container overnight.

Roasted Brussels Sprouts

SERVES 4

1½ pounds Brussels sprouts, trimmed and halved

2 tablespoons extra-virgin olive oil

Salt and freshly ground black pepper

2 tablespoons fresh lemon juice

2 tablespoons chopped fresh mint leaves

1. Preheat the oven to 450°F.

2. Combine the Brussels sprouts, oil, and a pinch each of salt and pepper in a large rimmed baking sheet. Toss until evenly coated.

3. Roast, stirring occasionally, until tender and browned, about 20 minutes.

4. Transfer to a large serving bowl and toss with the lemon juice and mint.

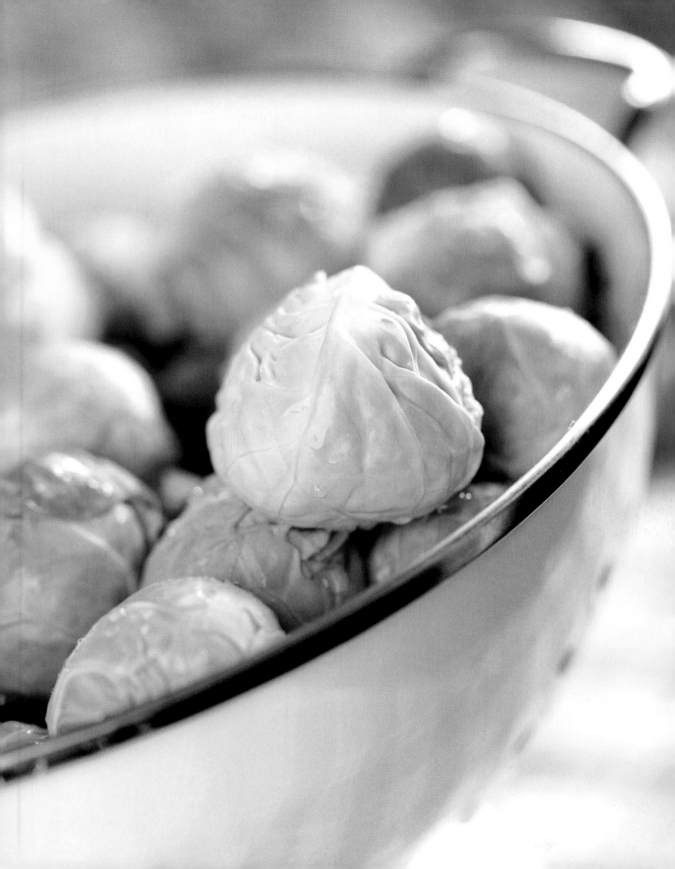

Roasted Mushrooms with Shallots and Parsley

SERVES 4

2 tablespoons extra-virgin olive oil

2 tablespoons (¼ stick) butter

1 pound fresh mushrooms, preferably a mixture of white, cremini, and shiitake, trimmed and wiped clean, cut into 1-inch pieces

2 small shallots, thinly sliced

1 tablespoon chopped fresh flat-leaf parsley leaves

Salt and freshly ground pepper

1. Preheat the oven to 400°F.

2. Combine the oil and butter in a large rimmed baking sheet. Place in the oven and remove when the butter melts, about 5 minutes.

3. Carefully add the mushrooms, shallots, parsley, and a pinch each of salt and pepper. Gently stir until evenly coated. Roast, stirring occasionally, until the mushrooms are golden brown, about 20 minutes.

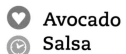

Avocado Salsa

MAKES ABOUT 7 CUPS

1²/₃ cups fresh corn kernels

1 cup ripe olives, sliced

1 red bell pepper, stemmed, seeded, and finely chopped

1 small onion, finely chopped

¼ cup fresh lemon juice

3 tablespoons cider vinegar

2 tablespoons extra-virgin olive oil

1 tablespoon chopped fresh oregano leaves

1 tablespoon chopped fresh cilantro leaves

Salt and freshly ground black pepper

4 ripe avocados

Tortilla chips, for serving

1. Combine the corn, olives, pepper, onion, lemon juice, vinegar, oil, oregano, and cilantro in a large bowl. Stir until well mixed. Season to taste with salt and pepper. Cover and refrigerate overnight.

2. Pit, peel, and chop the avocados. Gently fold into the corn mixture. Serve with tortilla chips.

Black Bean Salsa

SERVES 4

1 15-ounce can black beans, rinsed and drained

1 15-ounce can white corn, rinsed and drained

1 10-ounce can diced tomatoes with chiles

4 green onions, chopped

½ cup chopped fresh cilantro

1 tablespoon fresh lemon juice

2 tablespoons extra-virgin olive oil

Salt and freshly ground black pepper

1. Combine the black beans, corn, tomatoes, green onions, cilantro, lemon juice, oil, and a pinch each of salt and pepper.

2. Cover and refrigerate until cold, up to overnight. Serve with grilled fish.

Corn Bread from La Leche League Baking Mix

SERVES 6

1½ cups La Leche League Baking Mix (page 97)

¾ cup yellow cornmeal

1 tablespoon honey

1 large egg, beaten

1 cup whole milk

1. Preheat the oven to 400°F. Grease an 8-inch square cake pan.

2. Combine the baking mix, cornmeal, and honey in a large bowl. Stir in the egg and milk until the dry ingredients are moistened. Pour into the prepared pan.

3. Bake until golden and a toothpick inserted in the center comes out clean, 25 to 30 minutes.

4. Let cool in the pan on a wire rack. Serve warm.

Apple Bran Muffins

MAKES 1 DOZEN

1 cup whole-wheat flour

¾ cup wheat bran

¾ cup packed brown sugar

1½ teaspoons baking powder

¾ teaspoon baking soda

½ teaspoon cinnamon

½ teaspoon salt

½ cup canola oil

⅓ cup unsweetened applesauce

2 large eggs

¾ cup finely diced Granny Smith apple

½ cup golden raisins

1. Preheat the oven to 375°F. Line a muffin tin with paper liners.

2. Whisk together the flour, bran, sugar, baking powder, baking soda, cinnamon, and salt in a medium bowl.

3. Whisk together the oil, applesauce, and eggs in a large bowl until well blended. Add the flour mixture and stir until just blended. Fold in the apple and raisins.

4. Divide the batter among the prepared muffin cups. Bake until browned and a toothpick inserted in the center of one comes out clean, about 25 minutes.

5. Let cool in the pan on a wire rack for 5 minutes, then remove from the pan and cool completely on the wire rack.

Three Bears Porridge

SERVES 6

3 cups water or milk

½ cup cracked wheat

½ cup old-fashioned (rolled) oats

¼ cup oat bran

¼ cup wheat germ

¼ cup dry milk powder

¼ cup raisins

¼ cup chopped apple

½ teaspoon ground cinnamon

Honey, optional

½ cup sunflower seeds

1. Bring the water or milk to a boil in a large saucepan over high heat. Stir in the cracked wheat, oats, bran, wheat germ, milk powder, raisins, apple, and cinnamon. Reduce the heat to medium low, cover, and simmer, stirring occasionally, until thickened and cooked through, about 15 minutes.

2. Sweeten to taste with honey. Sprinkle sunflower seeds on top.

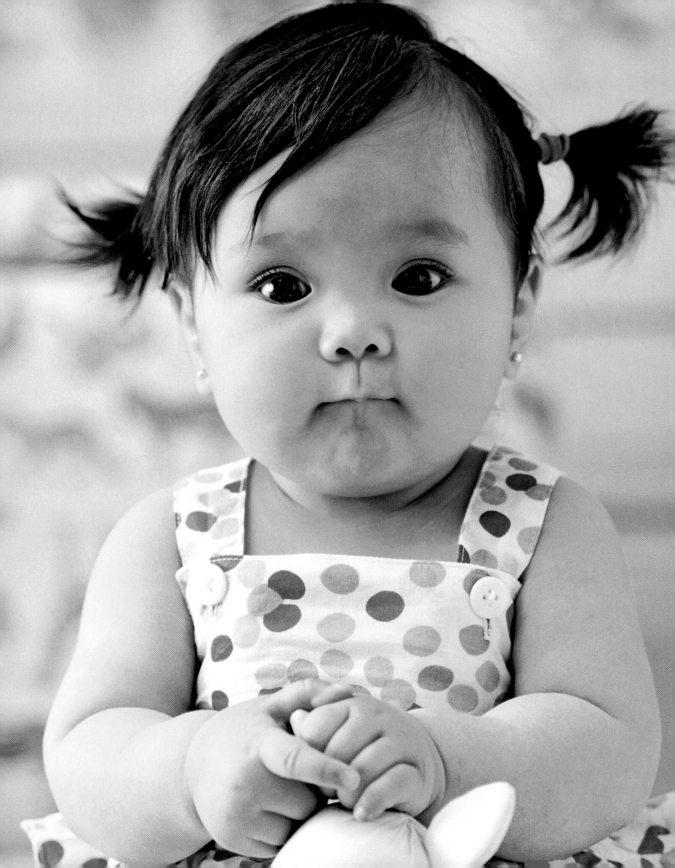

Chapter 4

Whole Foods for the Whole Family

FROM 6 TO 12 MONTHS

By now you're firmly "in the zone" with breastfeeding, and the early challenges of the first days, weeks, and months have vanished. You may have encountered a bout with the four-month fussies, when curious babies, stimulated by their environment, don't focus with their previous intensity on eating. Perhaps they nurse, stop to look around, "talk" about what they see and hear, and then go back to work—every 90 seconds. This phase passes, however, as your nursling matures beyond this distractible phase and gets back to the vital, nourishing business of eating. She is now very alert while she feeds, even as she looks into your eyes and relaxes by patting your breast, reaching up to touch your face, or simply grasping your fingers.

All her activity may make it harder for you to take in that healthy one-handed snack or meal while you nurse, but on the other hand, now it's easier to get a little time to yourself to sit at the table three times a day. In fact, at some point during this phase, she'll start to keep you company at mealtime—probably on your lap to start, and then, when she can sit up on her own (for many babies, at about 6 months or so), in a high chair or other safe seating arrangement beside you and the rest of her family.

Is she ready for solids? Let her lead the way, as you'll gradually and naturally learn to balance solids and nursing. You'll have plenty of time to ease into this new phase, as it will be well after her first birthday before she starts to favor solids over your milk.

Your diet and your baby's will continue to be intertwined, even as you approach the solid foods stage. During pregnancy, you were cautious about the foods you ate because you were protecting your unborn child, and you were eating carefully to stay healthy. After your child was born and breastfeeding began, your vigilance continued; you knew that what you ate would enter into your milk and that your baby might consume it in some form as well.

With breastfeeding established as the primary source of your child's nutrition, your attention to diet remains important—not just for her but for your own continued good health, energy, and well-being. And now, as she may eventually begin to show interest in some solid foods, your diet choices are still important. What you prepare for breakfast, lunch, or dinner; what you keep in the refrigerator and pantry; what you choose to snack on—it all matters to your baby because at some point she may be reaching for that food on your plate!

She may not eat any of it (it could be that shiny spoon she's after), or she may taste some banana or avocado and want more. Her interest may be piqued at around 6 months (or even earlier), or she may not have any curiosity or appetite for solids until much later. She may want it one day and feed it to the floor the next. No matter when it happens or how it happens, be ready with healthy and wholesome foods that you can share. As with breastfeeding, she is still eating what you eat.

"Watch your baby and not the calendar."

Eating Well So That Your Baby Will, Too

When you chose breastfeeding, you chose an excellent nutritional path for your child. Through your milk, he is protected from disease, allergens, obesity, and so much more. As an added bonus, if your diet is wide-ranging and healthful, he is exposed to a variety of tastes through your milk, ranging from savory to sweet to spicy to mellow. When you eat a varied diet and nurse, you are laying an excellent foundation for raising an agreeable and adventurous eater.

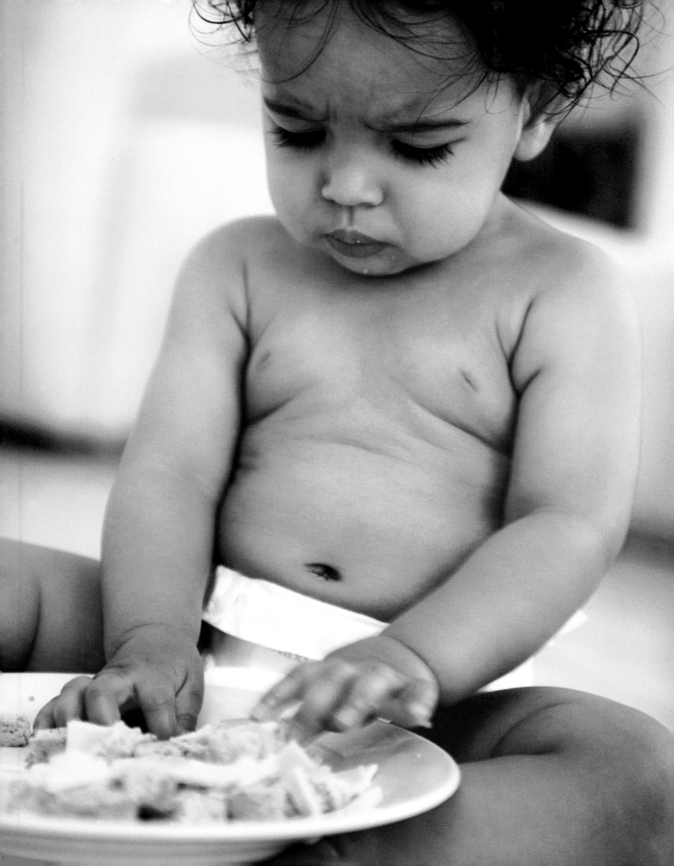

You should continue to consume healthy and balanced amounts of protein, calcium, iron, fiber, and folate. Interestingly, your daily calorie needs may increase slightly at about the 6-month mark, to around 400 extra calories per day (up from the 350 extra recommended on page 6).

One reason for this increase is that new mothers have a natural surplus of maternal fat stores they can tap in the early weeks and months. However, after 6 months of normal breastfeeding, these fat stores become depleted. Even though a baby may feed less frequently than he did as a newborn and infant, particularly in the second half of his first year, when complementary foods may be introduced, the maternal fat stores have now been used up; therefore, starting at around 6 months a breastfeeding mother generally needs these extra calories to support the next phase of lactation. (If she is ready to lose weight, keeping her calories at the same level—not adding the extra—is safe and will not impact breastfeeding.)

If you are working, your mealtimes—particularly breakfast and lunch—have probably reasserted themselves into your daily schedule at fairly predictable times, simply out of necessity. If you are at home and your day is more fluid, you may still be catching meals when it's convenient. Avoid falling into a pattern of eating too little or too late and then overeating at your next meal. For instance, it's very easy to overcompensate for no breakfast by overeating at lunch, because you are starving! Keep aiming for a balanced and varied diet, and if the evening meal is when you and your family come together at the table, continue to find ways to make the dinner hour less of a stress-fest and more of a way to wind down.

It's 6:00 p.m.—Do You Know Where Your Dinner Is?

The sun is lower in the sky and your nursling is in a good mood now, but he needs to be fed soon or else his coos will turn to cries. Your older child is hungry, too, for dinner and your attention. Your partner got stuck at work and will be even more famished than you are once the evening meal makes it to the table. It's time to nurse your baby and feed her sibling, plus two soon-to-be-starving adults, so you hit the panic button and order a pizza (again). But you know you should really be feeding yourself—and your family—with better choices. Consider these ideas the next time dinner threatens to undo you:

Slow-Cook It

The humble slow cooker is a time- and sanity-saver for many a family. The 1970s-era appliance has been updated and upgraded so that it's easy to clean and safer to use. Start a meal in the morning, when you have more time, and it's ready in the evening, when you're pressed. Best of all, the slow cooker shines when it comes to transforming healthy ingredients—vegetables, beans, meats, and other proteins cooked in low-fat, low-sodium broths—into hearty and satisfying meals. You'll find up-to-date recipes (beyond your mom's fondue or pot roast) in specialty slow cooker cookbooks; there are even websites dedicated to the resurgence of this "new" old appliance.

See our recipes for Slow Cooker Chuck Roast with Carrots, Tomatoes, and Potatoes (page 177), Slow Cooker Spinach Lasagna (page 84), Slow Cooker Vegetarian Chili (page 136), and Slow Cooker Split Pea Soup (page 182).

Lay In the Leftovers

Double up on main dishes or sides over the weekend or whenever you have time, and you'll be happier on a weeknight. If you're roasting one pork tenderloin, why not roast two? If you're making your favorite veggie chili, make some extra and freeze it.

Grill enough fish for two meals, bake extra muffins, cook extra brown rice. (See below for tips on freezing.) Cooked vegetables or dressed salads can lose their crunch and flavor, but most items will keep for a bit. Leftovers get a bad rap, but we're not talking about three-day-old limp broccoli or a cold, half-eaten burger. Good, nutritious food, set aside for second or third meals, becomes great food when you need a home-cooked meal on the table in the time it takes to open the fridge and reheat.

It's 6:00 p.m.—Do You Know Where Your Dinner Is? (CONTINUED)

Freeze It

Experiment with what freezes well, and get into the habit of keeping your freezer well stocked with precooked meal makings. Soups, stews, casseroles, cooked beans, and many baked pastas freeze very well. Whole grains such as brown rice can be cooked, then cooled, frozen in plastic bags (lay them flat), and reheated as needed (microwave, or thaw and reheat on the stove). Most baked goods and savory pies such as main-dish quiches freeze nicely. (Cooked pancakes or waffles can be frozen individually, wrapped in plastic. To reheat, remove from the plastic, place in foil, and bake at 350°F for 8–10 minutes, or as you wish.) Even some staples, such as butter, can be frozen.

Why pay for commercially frozen foods, often highly processed and full of additives you and your family don't need, when you can make it and freeze it yourself? For more information on how to safely freeze and reheat cooked and uncooked foods, visit the USDA's website for the following fact sheet: www.fsis.usda.gov/factsheets/focus_on_freezing.

For a complete list of recipes in this book that are freezer-friendly, see pages 79–81.

Order It

If you do call for the pizza or the take-out of your choice (and it happens to most of us at some point), add a large side salad and fruit for dessert and it becomes more balanced. If you have to fall back on prepared food, keep it as basic as possible—such as the fully cooked rotisserie chicken from the market, which has rescued many a mom (and dad), or a veggie pizza with a whole-grain crust.

But here's another ordering tip: take advantage of online grocery ordering and delivery. Many websites and grocery store chains, and even some smaller food markets, allow you to shop online and get your staples (and fresh items) delivered; you can also go low-tech with stores that allow you to place a phone order the old-fashioned way. We have already discussed the importance of filling the refrigerator, freezer, and pantry with the good stuff (see the lists on pages 18–22) so that you're never caught off-guard for healthy meals and snacks. The trick is keeping the larder stocked.

Ask for It

Finally, if you work and have in-home child care, and if your caregiver is amenable, ask if she'd be willing to chop some ingredients ahead of time, start reheating whatever is on the menu, or just turn the oven on by a certain time. This small task will save you precious minutes when you walk through the door. If your partner works, too, plan menus together in advance, particularly if you often arrive home at different times. Food prep (or just getting a jump on reheating) can be time-consuming, but work is cut in half when your partner helps, leaving you more time to relax as a family. (For a list of make-ahead recipes, see pages 217–18.) ▪

Good Food for Good Health: Our "Whole Foods for the Whole Family" Approach

It's difficult not to be tempted by the numerous mealtime shortcuts that are marketed to busy parents. You can simply open a box, add water, microwave for a couple of minutes, and dinner is served. But if you've been reading the labels and trying to limit items such as trans fat and sodium, you know that such packaged, processed foods are rarely, if ever, the best choices. You may save time, but nutritionally, the price can be quite high. And many times, packaged foods promoted as economical and quick solutions are neither inexpensive nor significantly time-saving.

At La Leche League International, we embraced the message of "whole foods for the whole family" decades ago, when we celebrated the idea of recipes based on natural ingredients and unprocessed foods—items such as whole grains; fresh fruits and vegetables; good-quality meat, fish, poultry, and dairy; no hydrogenated fats or preservatives—in our cookbook of the same name

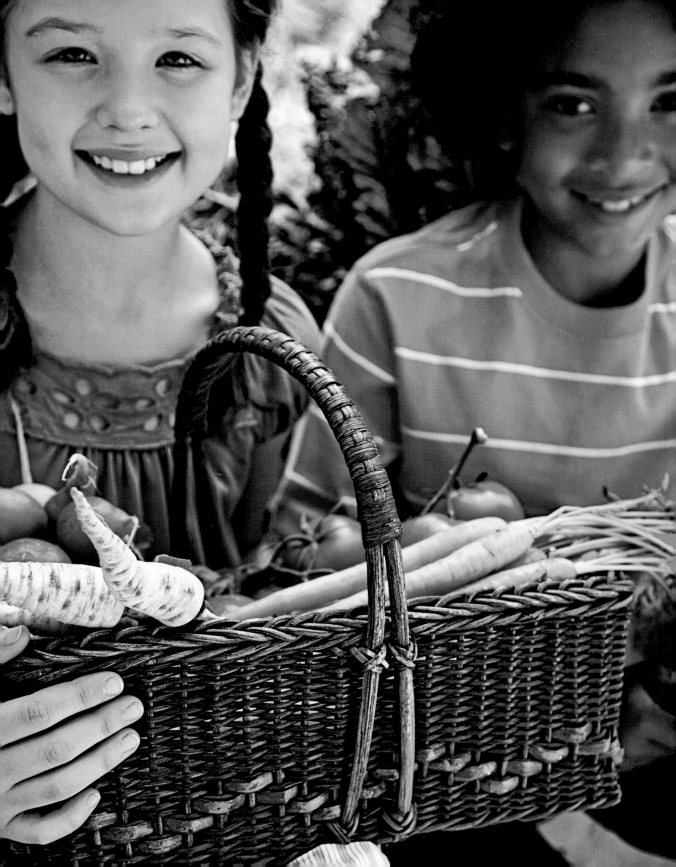

(**Whole Foods for the Whole Family**, first published in 1981). This reflects the LLLI definition of good nutrition, which we mentioned earlier: a well-balanced and varied diet of foods in as close to their natural state as possible.

Today, families no longer need to belong to specialty food co-ops or shop at tiny health food stores to purchase items such as whole-wheat pasta or organic produce. Large supermarket chains offer a range of affordable, healthy foods (plenty of them organic), and in recent years local farmer's markets have flourished in many communities, big and small. (See page 70 for more information on the Community Supported Agriculture concept and how it can benefit your family.)

There is an abundance of good food available, but still, making healthy choices remains challenging for many. Obesity rates and weight-related health problems (such as heart disease and diabetes) among adults and children are alarming, and food manufacturers continue to manufacture and market unhealthy foods and beverages—directly to kids, in many instances—because they are highly lucrative products.

If your baby is less than a year old, even if he has begun taking solid foods, your milk is still his main source of nourishment, and thinking about his diet in terms of junk food versus real food may seem, well, unpalatable. However, it's not too early to think about how to raise a healthy eater who will make wise choices into adulthood.

"He ate what we ate. And we ate considerably better after he began solids."

You can set the tone now, by making the very best choices for yourself and keeping your kitchen filled with good food. You may already have an excellent and well-balanced diet, or you may—like many of us—have a few areas that need some fine-tuning (perhaps in the areas we're about to address). If you yourself embrace the "whole foods for the whole family" way of eating, you will make that pathway clearer for your child.

Sweet and Savory: How to Season Your Whole-Foods Diet

You may already have highly processed or high-fat items on your grocery store radar as things to avoid, not good for you and not good for your children. So you skip the big-brand boxed macaroni and cheese and reach for the organic version; you buy low-fat baked pita chips instead of greasy potato chips; you purchase frozen yogurt instead of butter pecan ice cream; you put whole-wheat sandwich bread and natural peanut butter in your basket. All these foods and products meet your whole-foods criteria, and you feel pretty confident about what's in the cart as you check out.

If you're shopping this way, you're clearly interested in making the best choices. Still, we'd like to zero in on two common ingredients that appear in many (if not all) of those healthy foods you've selected, and which are easy to overconsume because they are so ubiquitous. As you look to feeding your whole family—including a future eater of table food—and not just yourself, be mindful of two everyday substances that appear on our plates in some form each day: salt and sugar.

Salt: Shake It Easy

Iodized table salt contains iodine, a trace element that all humans need in order to synthesize thyroid hormones, which regulate metabolism and allow for normal growth. Adults need 150 micrograms; pregnant women need 220 micrograms; breastfeeding women need slightly more, 290 micrograms. (Not all salt is iodized. Sea salt generally has less iodine—about one-tenth that of iodized table salt. And kosher salt usually does not contain iodine.)

Iodized table salt is an extremely concentrated iodine source; ¼ teaspoon will give you 100 micrograms. You needn't consume much iodized table salt to get the iodine you need. Iodine also exists naturally in saltwater fish and shellfish such as clams, lobsters, oysters, sardines, and other seafood. It can be found in milk and eggs, and some foods made with them (such as certain breads), because cows and chickens are given feed containing iodine. Some fruits and vegetables, including potatoes, also contain iodine if they are grown in iodine-rich soil. Because of the introduction of iodized table salt and its use in commonly consumed foods, iodine deficiency (and its results, such as an enlarged thyroid gland or goiter) is not a common health concern for most of us, though it remains a public health problem in many parts of the world.

You also don't need much table salt for another reason: too much sodium is harmful to us. The body needs sodium to maintain a proper fluid balance and for nerve and muscle function, among other things, but excess sodium can lead to serious health problems, including high blood pressure and heart disease—even in children.

The latest USDA dietary guidelines suggest that healthy adults eat no more than 2,300 milligrams of salt per day; children, African Americans, people over 50, and those with hypertension, diabetes, or chronic kidney disease should have no more than 1,500 milligrams. Just to put that into perspective, **1 teaspoon** of table salt has a whole day's worth of sodium for a healthy adult. Furthermore, these guidelines are set as the upper limits of what we should be consuming. Studies show that many American adults actually consume about 3,400 milligrams per day.

To be clear, our population's overconsumption of sodium is largely attributed to consumption of processed and prepared food—restaurant food, frozen dinners, packaged deli meats, chips and pretzels, boxed rice or pasta mixes, canned goods, condiments such as soy sauce, and much more. It is estimated that about 75 percent of the sodium we take in comes from such foods.[1] If you are shopping smartly and avoiding highly processed foods, then you and your family should be safe from too much sodium, right? The problem is that even healthy foods may contribute to taking in more sodium than we need. Whole-grain breakfast cereal, organic canned soups and vegetables, high-quality jarred pasta sauces (and the can of tomato sauce you buy to make your own pasta sauce), low-fat fresh deli turkey breast, nuts, multigrain crackers, calcium-rich cheese, and even a cup of low-fat milk—these healthy choices and many other good foods may not taste overly salted, but their sodium content can add up.

Your best bet is to be label-savvy and be mindful of the amounts of sodium in the foods you buy; scan ingredients for any version of the word "sodium," including the word "soda" (for baking soda and sodium bicarbonate), and the chemical symbol for sodium, Na. Note the serving sizes as well; many nutritionists recommend that a single serving of food should not exceed 300 milligrams of sodium.

Canned beans can be an excellent staple to keep at the ready, but buy no-salt-added, or rinse the beans before you use them. Look for no- or low-salt versions of soups, sauces, and dressings. (See the box on page 162 for what "low-salt" and other similar terms actually mean.) Salt your home-cooked foods **after** you taste-test. Better yet, experiment with spices, herbs, and lemon juice to flavor your savory foods and reduce salt. If you or your partner automatically reaches for the salt shaker at mealtime, take it off the dining table and put it back in the kitchen so that someone has to get up and retrieve it—and with that process think about how much you're adding to your diet.

If you think you're exceeding the normal level of sodium and you're breast-feeding, you won't harm your nursling with salty milk; fortunately, our bodies have multiple built-in balance systems that keep this from happening. If a breastfeeding mother (or any person, for that matter) consumes too much sodium, the body responds with a hormonal response in the kidneys that causes thirst. We drink; our bodies make urine to balance out the excess sodium; we urinate. However, if a breastfeeding mother is **severely** dehydrated with no access to fluids, the sodium in breast milk could become more concentrated. Fortunately, such dehydration is highly unlikely to happen under normal living conditions. Still, if you're eating too much salt, even if it doesn't affect your milk and your baby, you're compromising your own health.

So think about the littlest eater at the table, even if for now she's just there to play with a spoon and be with her family. "Remember that your baby does not know the taste of salt and does not crave salty food," Margaret Kenda writes in **Whole Foods for Babies and Toddlers**, one of our follow-ups to **Whole Foods for the Whole Family**.[2] "If you add salt to baby food, you may find it tastes better to you. But the baby will not eat better or find the food tastier."

Given the facts on the overconsumption of sodium, you will be contributing to your baby's good health—beyond childhood and into her adulthood—if you curb the salt. You'll also be helping yourself and the rest of your family.

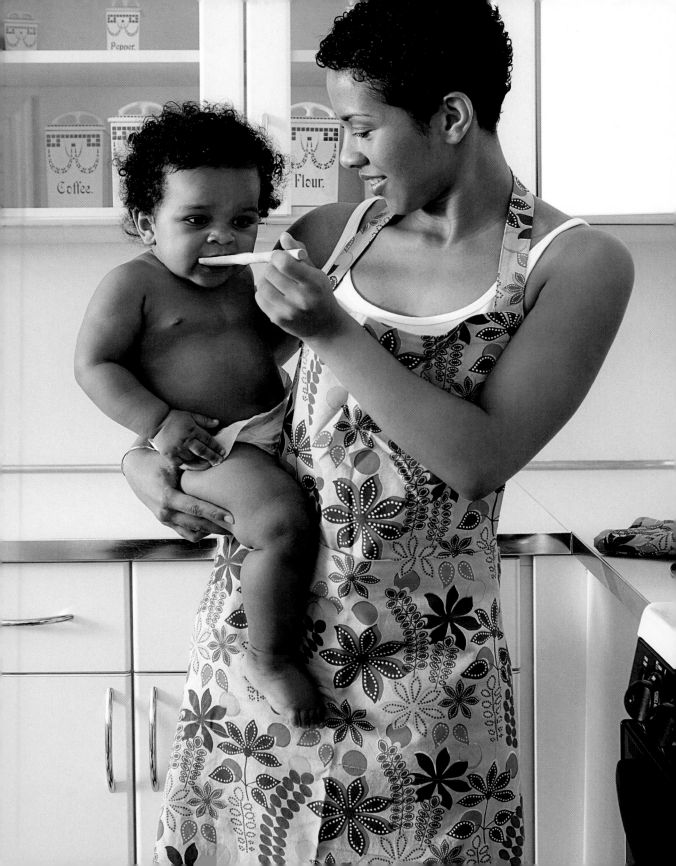

"How Much Salt Is in Here?" What the Labels Mean

If you're seeking out lower-sodium products, you'll encounter the following terms. Some sound similar (such as "reduced sodium" and "lightly salted"), but each has a different meaning.

Sodium free—less than 5 milligrams of sodium per serving

Very low sodium—35 milligrams or less per serving

Low sodium—140 milligrams or less per serving

Reduced sodium—usual sodium level is reduced by 25 percent

Lightly salted—usual sodium level is reduced by 50 percent

Healthy—does not exceed 480 milligrams sodium per serving if it's an individual food (such as beans); does not exceed 600 milligrams sodium per serving if it's a meal-type food (such as a frozen entrée)

Unsalted, no salt added, or without added salt—made without salt that's normally used, but still contains the sodium that's a natural part of the food itself[3]

Sugar: An Added Ingredient That Does Not Add Much

Whether a product label says sucrose, dextrose, fructose, corn syrup, honey, sorghum syrup, turbinado sugar, molasses, maltose, malted barley, maple syrup, brown sugar, raw sugar, organic cane juice/sugar, or other names you've probably seen, if it's on the ingredient list it's added sugar.

According to the USDA, the United States is the largest consumer of sweeteners, including high-fructose corn syrup, and one of the top global producers (and importers) of sugar. Sugar, added sugar, everywhere . . . and a lot of it winds up in our food supply, not just in obvious places such as low-nutrition, high-cal desserts, candy, and soda, but even creeping into some whole-grain bread products and cereals, low-fat yogurt, peanut butter, and other products we turn to when we're looking for healthy foods for ourselves and our families.

Sugar is a carbohydrate and we need carbohydrates in order to produce energy-making glucose (a form of sugar), which the body requires. (See pages 14–15 for more on the importance of carbohydrates.) Glucose fuels our system by circulating throughout the bloodstream and providing energy on a cellular level. To put it simply, when we have stable levels of glucose in our system, we feel pretty good. But as mentioned in Chapter 1, getting carbohydrates from sugar is ill advised because the bloodstream rapidly absorbs this simple carb for a burst of energy; the body naturally uses up the calories that simple sugar provides and our glucose levels rapidly get knocked out of balance, leaving us feeling depleted. This is why the best sources of energy-making carbohydrates are the complex carbs discussed in Chapter 1.

While different forms of added sugar could be considered more healthful than others (certainly "organic pure cane sugar" sounds more appealing than "high-fructose corn syrup"), be aware that **added sugar is sugar**, and no matter where it comes from, an excess will play havoc with your body's glucose levels.

Read and compare labels carefully, even on that fresh and wholesome-looking loaf of "honey whole-wheat" bread you're putting into your cart, and when your child is old enough, teach her to do the same. She'll probably have to contend with children's breakfast cereals, granola bars, yogurt, fruit leather, juice and juice drinks, flavored milks, and many other kid-friendly products that are regularly offered to children as "healthful" snacks but which often have unnecessary added sugars.

There are about 4 grams of sugar in 1 teaspoon; according to the Dietary Guidelines for Americans, we should limit our consumption to no more than 8 teaspoons total (32 grams) per day. That may sound like a lot, but consider that a low-fat flavored yogurt with 28 grams of sugar has the equivalent of 7 teaspoons—there goes most of the daily allowance. A 12-ounce can of cola has about 10 teaspoons. A "lightly sweetened" multigrain breakfast cereal with 12 grams of sugar per serving has 3 teaspoons. It's challenging to avoid the sugar in the foods we buy, but reading labels and being aware is an excellent first step. We can also make a difference when we prepare our own whole foods at home. A few suggestions:

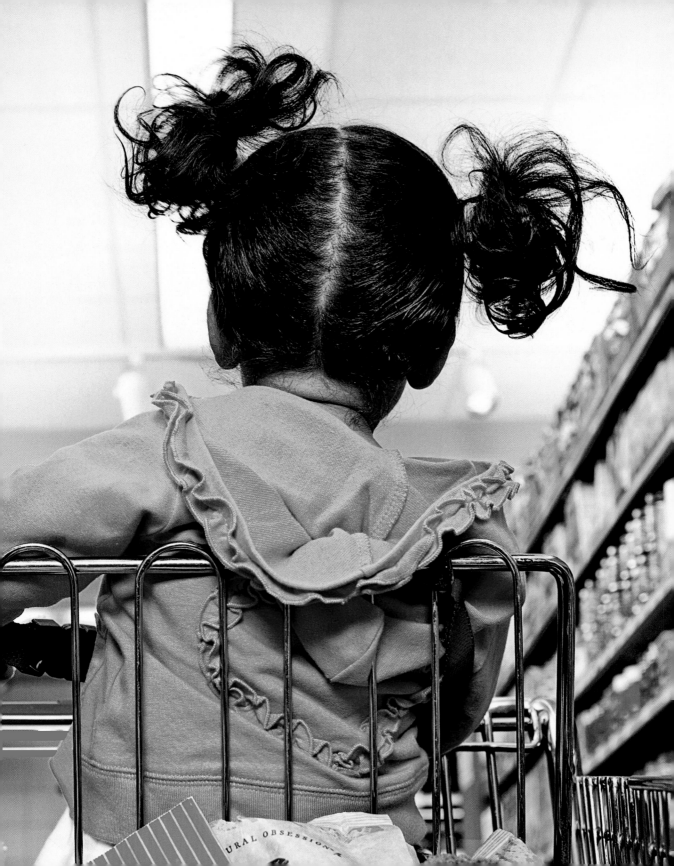

- Buy plain yogurt, not flavored, and sweeten it with your own fruit puree or chopped fruits.
- Top pancakes or waffles with fruit instead of syrup (a tablespoon of pure maple syrup has the equivalent of 3 teaspoons of sugar).
- Make your own granola to control the sugar (dried fruits can be healthful but high in sugar, so don't overdo it).
- Experiment with recipes—reduce the sugar and see if you taste a difference. Where appropriate, use spices such as cinnamon, vanilla, and nutmeg for flavor.
- Cut pure fruit juice with seltzer for a fizzy, not-too-sweet refreshment.

If you have a sweet tooth, try your best to tame it now, before your child is old enough to wonder why it's okay for you to drink the large soda while he has plain water. Though it is true that babies and young children do have a preference for sweet things, make sure they are getting that sweet taste from healthy sources such as fruits and vegetables, and don't let added sugars add empty calories to their diets, or yours. (If you're looking for a sweet but healthy treat, see the recipe for Dandy Candy, page 241, a La Leche League International favorite that has satisfied many a child—and many a grown-up, too!)

> "I let my son have some cake on his first birthday. Other than that we avoided all sugar and juice until after his second birthday. We were very conscious to make sure that all the sugar he got up until that point was fructose and that it came directly from fresh fruit. You can really tell the difference sugar makes in their behavior when you don't give them **any** and then they get some. Sugar is nobody's friend."

Taste Buds in Training: Your Baby's Developing Palate

All babies are different when it comes to solids, which is why we think baby-led feeding is the most natural approach. (See page 170 later in this chapter for more information on the baby-led approach.) Taking cues from your baby on when he wants to eat solid foods is an extension of breastfeeding on demand.

La Leche League International states: "For the healthy full-term baby breast milk is the only food necessary until baby shows signs of needing solids, about the middle of the first year after birth." Still, parents are routinely advised by pediatricians to start solids based on the oft-repeated "between 4 and 6 months" rule that appears in much of the medical and parenting literature. Four months is not a magical start date, nor is 6 months some kind of deadline. It is helpful to be aware of the important developmental reasons that cause this "window" to come up so frequently, and to be prepared to follow your baby's cues as to when they are ready to start solids.

At **1 month of age**, your nursling could suck, swallow, and breathe at the same time, as well as gag (a lifesaving reflex) and close her lips. **By 3 months**, she had added some head control.

At **4 months**, she had improved lip closure and increased tongue control; she was also starting to develop the beginnings of hand-to-mouth coordination. Her tongue-thrust reflex, which all babies are born with and which stops them from choking, possibly began to weaken. (Until this natural reflex diminishes, usually at about the 6-month mark, a baby will continue to push food out with her tongue, rather than taking it in for swallowing.) **At 5 months**, she exhibited a basic bite-and-release pattern. Her suckling and sucking continued, but she had increased oral sensitivity and teething may have begun. Her hand-to-mouth coordination improved, too. Now, at this point in your baby's life and looking ahead to her first birthday:

- **At 6 months**, she has good lip control, can extend and retract her tongue, and recognizes a spoon. This is why she might be interested in some very soft foods at this point. When food is placed on her lower lip, she will draw it inward. She is also starting to move her tongue from side to side.
- **At 7 months**, she can be fed in a sitting position. She can move her tongue horizontally to get at food in the side of her mouth.
- **At 8 months**, she can use her upper lip to remove food from a spoon. She is able to eat soft whole foods and mashed-up table food. Thanks to improved hand-to-mouth coordination and a developing grip, she can finger-feed.

- **At 9 months**, she can chew up and down and on a diagonal. She will hold a soft cookie or cracker between her gums without biting.
- **At 12 months**, she sucks liquid from a cup. Her jaw moves up and down and her lips may be open during swallowing. She can bite with whatever teeth she may have, and now can manage ground, mashed, or chopped table food with noticeable lumps. Her upper incisors help remove food from the lower lip, and she can transfer food to the sides of the mouth for chewing. She also will cough or choke if she eats too fast.

No two babies are alike, and they will not all reach these milestones on the same day. Still, it's useful to get a general picture of how their abilities to take in food develop, and to recognize the numerous physical reasons why La Leche League International recommends that "for the healthy full-term baby breast milk is the only food necessary until baby shows signs of needing solids, about the middle of the first year after birth."

What About Iron?

Though breast milk contains low levels of iron, it is the type of iron that is more completely absorbed by your baby than the kind of iron in formula, baby cereal, or iron supplements. Even if a baby is exclusively breastfed, her pediatrician, if he is following the latest recommendations from the AAP and other health organizations, may recommend supplementary iron (in drop form) around 4 months of age, particularly if baby has not started on solids. Seek out iron-rich foods such as meats, dark green leafy vegetables, and beets.

Depending on the soil these foods are grown in, they can be high in naturally occurring nitrates, which could cause a form of anemia. Commercial baby food made with these vegetables is considered safe because manufacturers screen produce they purchase for nitrates. The AAP suggests waiting one year before offering home-prepared versions of spinach, beets, turnips, carrots, or collard greens in their brochure "Starting

> **What About Iron?** (CONTINUED)
>
> Solid Foods" (2008); other sources, such as the Mayo Clinic, state that they can be given after 4 months. Nitrate poisoning from contaminated vegetables is extremely rare and stems from contaminated soil. Check with your pediatrician for the latest guidelines. ▪

Food Allergies and Sensitivities

Even if you or your baby's father has no history of food allergies, you may be wondering about whether your nursling will at some point develop a food allergy or sensitivity. Food allergies and sensitivities are a common topic and source of concern among many parents, in part because some studies suggest that they are on the rise. (Peanut allergies, for instance, are being diagnosed at a higher rate than they were in previous generations.) In a study conducted by Scott H. Sicherer, M.D., a pediatrician and food allergy expert, researchers noted an increase of nut allergies in children, from 4 per 1,000 in 1997 to 8 per 1,000 in 2003—a 100 percent increase. Though some experts suggest that peanut butter not be given before age 2 (in children with a parent who has a peanut allergy, the recommendation is not before age 3), this recommendation is now being questioned by many pediatric allergy researchers and experts. (For instance, as of 2008 the AAP no longer stipulated the waiting period for peanut products.)

The most allergenic foods for children are milk, eggs, soy, peanuts, wheat, fish, and shellfish. If given too early, when the intestinal lining is not mature, there is a higher risk of a reaction. (See pages 126–28.) "The gut is much more permeable before four months, so whole proteins can be absorbed easily, which increases the risk of developing an allergy," says William Dietz, M.D., director of the division of nutrition and physical activity at the Centers for Disease Control and Prevention in Atlanta.[4]

However, there are no conclusive studies about whether or not these foods should be withheld as first foods in order to reduce the risk of allergy or sensitivity. The American Academy of Pediatrics, for instance, points out that fish and eggs have often been on the "not yet" list among many pediatricians, but they also happen to be healthful foods that offer benefits to a growing baby who is starting solids.

Many experts in childhood nutrition recommend introducing one new food at a time, waiting two or three days before introducing another. Stop the new food and consult with your pediatrician if your baby reacts with vomiting, diarrhea, rash, or other unusual symptoms that could signal allergy or sensitivity.

If you or your baby's father has food allergies, your approach to solids will understandably be more cautious than that in an allergy-free household, and you'll want to work with your health care provider to determine best practices for introducing your child to solids. Though your baby has an increased risk of allergy due to genetic factors, the development of allergy is not a sure thing.

As you move into this phase and determine the best start time for your nursling, do so with the confidence that breastfeeding is one of the most effective ways to continue protecting your child against food allergies and sensitivities—the protective effects carry on into adolescence. So keep doing what you're doing, particularly when the time comes to introduce solids.

First Foods: From Thin to Thick, from Soft to Less Soft (but Not Hard!)

At the end of this section, you'll find a list of "starter foods," originally developed for and published in **The Womanly Art of Breastfeeding**. If you review the information earlier in this chapter (see pages 165–67) on how a baby develops the physical capability to eat solids, you'll recognize that not all foods on this list are equal in terms of texture. A ripe banana, for instance, is mushy and soft; a whole-wheat breadstick is harder (though when baby gums it in his mouth he's sure to make it mushy and soft). Keep in mind that texture matters to a new eater. He is learning to use his tongue to move food side to side, closing his lips, and chewing up and down and diagonally. Each food is a new adventure, and some may be more challenging than others. With that in mind, use the list of starter foods to get ideas; use the information that follows to determine when baby might be ready for new textures.

> **About 6 months to 8 months:** Soft, smooth table foods (no mixed textures yet)
>
> **9 months:** Hard foods that melt or dissolve (graham crackers, frozen fruit chunks)
>
> **10 months:** Soft cubes (avocado, soft cooked squash, potatoes)
>
> **11 months:** Soft chewables with a single texture (very thin slices of meat, scrambled eggs, pasta)
>
> **12 months:** Soft chewables with mixed textures (moist chicken pieces, macaroni and cheese, baked sweet potato fries (see our recipe page 238), spaghetti with meat sauce)

Baby-Led: A Natural Approach

La Leche League International recommends letting baby lead the way when it comes to weaning and starting solids, saying that "ideally the breastfeeding relationship will continue until the baby outgrows the need." This philosophy, often referred to as baby-led weaning, promotes self-feeding of appropriate foods in safe sizes and shapes.[5] For instance, instead of pureed, jarred banana baby food fed to a baby with a spoon, a baby can be offered soft, baby-fist-size chunks of banana that she will feed to herself. She can experience the pure taste of whole foods through the baby-led approach and will set the pace of how much she wants to eat. The baby-led way is a natural complement to breastfeeding, promotes independence in eating, and helps your child to develop a healthy relationship with food. More information on starting solids can be found in Chapter 13 of **The Womanly Art of Breastfeeding,** 8th edition. ◼

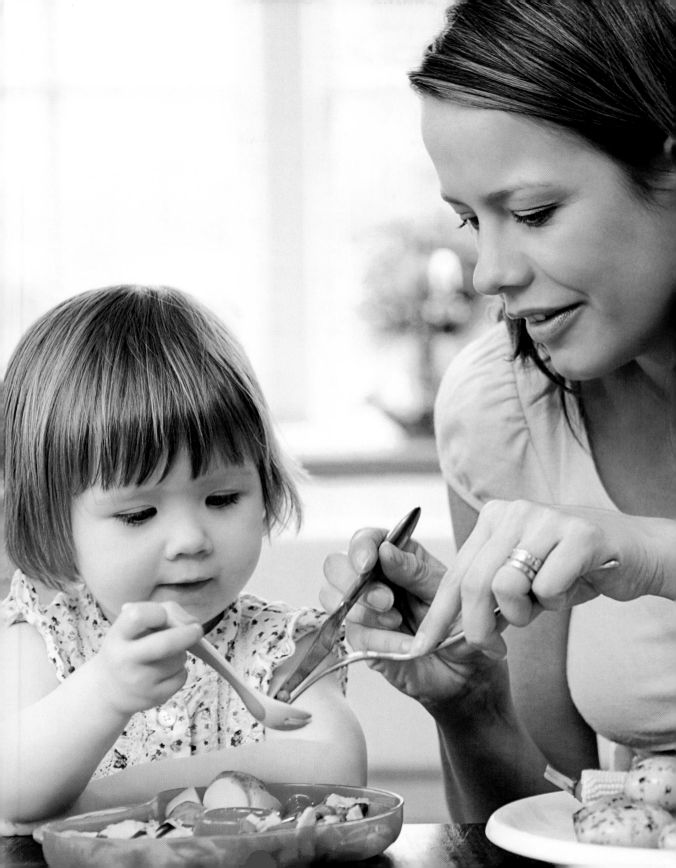

FAVORITE FOODS IN THE FIRST YEAR

Fruits: slightly mushy or baby-fist-size chunks to hold

Apple—peeled, grated, or lightly cooked
Avocado
Banana
Blueberries—frozen or raw
Melon
Pear

Meats: cooked (shredded or slivered) versions to gnaw on

Chicken—remove the bone, or offer a drumstick with just a little meat still
  on the bone
Fish—serve small pieces of flaky well-cooked fish; watch for bones
Ground beef, pork, or lamb; or offer a bone from beef, pork, or lamb with
  fat and most meat removed

Vegetables: cooked till limp or cooked and mashed

Beans—very soft or mashed
Carrots—very soft or mashed (see note pages 167–68 on nitrates)
Hummus—try offering it on your finger
Peas—frozen or cooked; removing skins helps digestion
String beans
Sweet potato—big chunk or mashed with water or breast milk
White potato—big chunk or mashed with water or your milk

Grains

Rice cakes
Sticky rice
Whole-grain breads (stale for gnawing)
Whole-wheat breadsticks

Proteins and Fats for the Vegan/Vegetarian Baby*

Avocados (fat source: avocados contain no protein)
Beans and lentils, very soft or mashed
Nut butters (for nonallergic families)
Seed butters (such as tahini) as dips or spreads
Seitan

If a food is traditional for babies in your family, and if your baby is old enough, go for it!

FOODS ASSOCIATED WITH ALLERGY, RASH, AND FOOD SENSITIVITY

Berries containing small, hard seeds (such as strawberries, raspberries, and blackberries)
Citrus fruits (including oranges, lemons, and grapefruit)
Corn products
Cow milk and dairy products (maybe the most common allergens)
Egg whites (yolks generally okay)
Kiwi
Peanuts and peanut butter
Shellfish

CHOKING RISKS: NOT SUITABLE FOR BABIES AND TODDLERS

Hot dogs, even small slices
Nuts
Popcorn

* If you are raising your baby vegan, don't forget his need for supplementary vitamin B_{12}; talk to your doctor if you have any concerns.

Raw carrots and similar hard foods
Whole grapes

OTHER PROBLEM FOODS TO AVOID

Dried fruits, including raisins, dates, and figs—too sticky for them to deal with easily

Foods high in saturated fat, such as fried foods—unhealthy, hard to digest

Foods high in salt—unhealthy

Foods that contain added sugar or artificial sweeteners—unhealthy

Honey or corn syrup—may contain botulism spores, which you can handle but a baby under 1 can't

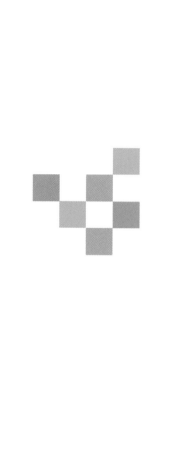

Veggie and Beef Meatloaf

SERVES 4

1 tablespoon extra-virgin olive oil, plus more for pan

1 large onion, finely chopped

3 carrots, finely diced

Salt and freshly ground black pepper

4 cups baby spinach

½ cup plain dry bread crumbs

¼ cup reduced-fat (2%) milk

1 large egg

1 teaspoon Worcestershire sauce

¼ cup plus 2 tablespoons ketchup

1 pound ground lean beef

1. Preheat the oven to 350°F. Line a rimmed baking sheet with foil and lightly grease the foil.

2. Heat the oil in a large skillet over medium heat. Add the onion, carrots, 3 tablespoons water, and a pinch each of salt and pepper. Cover and cook, stirring occasionally, until very tender, about 10 minutes. Stir in the spinach and cook until just wilted, about 1 minute. Remove from the heat and transfer to cutting board. When cool enough to handle, finely chop.

3. Meanwhile, combine the bread crumbs and milk in a large bowl and let stand for 5 minutes. Add the egg, Worcestershire sauce, and 2 tablespoons ketchup, and mix with a fork. Add the beef and the vegetable mixture. Gently mix until well combined.

4. Transfer the meat mixture to the prepared pan and shape into a rectangular 8-by-4-inch loaf. Spread the remaining ¼ cup ketchup over the top.

5. Bake until cooked through, about 1 hour.

Slow Cooker Chuck Roast with Carrots, Tomatoes, and Potatoes

SERVES 6

6 carrots, cut into 2-inch pieces

4 red potatoes, cut into 1-inch chunks

3 celery stalks, cut into 1-inch pieces

2 large onions, sliced

2 fresh thyme sprigs

1 dried bay leaf

1 tablespoon cornstarch

Salt and freshly ground black pepper

1 14.5-ounce can diced tomatoes

1 2½-pound beef chuck roast

1. Combine the carrots, potatoes, celery, onions, thyme, bay leaf, cornstarch, and a pinch each of salt and pepper in the bowl of a 5½-quart slow cooker. Toss until evenly coated, then spread in an even layer. Pour the tomatoes over.

2. Sprinkle salt and pepper all over the chuck roast. Place on top of the vegetables. Cover and cook on low for 8 hours or on high for 5 hours. It is done when the meat is fork tender and the vegetables are tender.

3. Transfer the roast to a cutting board and cut into slices across the grain. Serve with the vegetables and pan juices.

Baked Salmon with Apricot Glaze

SERVES 4

3 tablespoons lower-sodium soy sauce

3 tablespoons apricot jam

2 tablespoons peeled and grated fresh ginger

½ teaspoon fresh lemon zest

4 6-ounce skinless center-cut salmon fillets

1. Preheat the oven to 350°F.

2. Stir the soy sauce, jam, ginger, and lemon zest in a large baking dish until well mixed. Add the salmon and turn until evenly coated with the glaze. Spoon any remaining glaze over the tops of the salmon fillets.

3. Bake the salmon until just opaque throughout, about 12 minutes. A knife will pierce easily through the flesh.

Broccoli Pesto Multigrain Pasta

SERVES 6

1 lemon

1 pound broccoli florets

1 box (13 to 14 ounces) whole-grain penne or spaghetti

1 cup packed fresh basil leaves

Salt and freshly ground black pepper

¼ cup extra-virgin olive oil

⅓ cup freshly grated Parmesan cheese

1. Bring a large pot of water to a boil.

2. Meanwhile, zest the lemon into a food processor and squeeze 2 tablespoons juice over.

3. Add the broccoli to the boiling water and cook, stirring occasionally, until bright green and just tender, about 5 minutes. Use a slotted spoon to transfer the broccoli to the food processor.

4. Return the water to a boil and add the pasta to the same pot. Cook according to the package directions. Reserve ¼ cup cooking water.

5. Add the basil and a pinch each of salt and pepper to the food processor. Process until finely chopped. With the machine running, add the oil and then the reserved pasta cooking water.

6. Drain the pasta and return to the pot. Add the broccoli pesto and toss until evenly coated. Season to taste with salt and pepper.

Summer Squash Omelets

SERVES 4

3 tablespoons extra-virgin olive oil

1 yellow summer squash, trimmed and diced

Salt and freshly ground black pepper

2 cups baby spinach

1 medium plum tomato, cored, seeded, and diced

2 ounces pasteurized goat cheese, crumbled

8 large eggs

1. Preheat the oven to 200°F.

2. Heat 1 tablespoon oil in a small nonstick skillet on medium-high. Add the squash, sprinkle with salt and pepper, and cook, stirring occasionally, until browned and just tender, about 3 minutes. Add the spinach and cook, stirring, just until wilted, about 1 minute. Transfer to bowl and add tomato and cheese, stirring to mix.

3. Beat the eggs with a pinch each of salt and pepper until just blended.

4. Wipe out the skillet, then heat 1½ teaspoons oil in it on medium. When the oil is hot, pour one-quarter of the eggs into the skillet. When the edges begin to set, use a spatula to lift the cooked edges to let the uncooked egg run underneath. When the bottom is evenly set but the top is still moist, sprinkle one-quarter of the tomato, cheese, and squash mixture over half of the eggs. Use the spatula to fold the unfilled half over the filled side.

5. Slide onto an ovenproof plate and keep warm in the oven. Repeat with the remaining eggs and filling.

Soft Scrambled Eggs with Leeks

SERVES 4

1 leek, white and pale green parts only, halved lengthwise and thinly sliced crosswise

2 tablespoons extra-virgin olive oil

Salt and freshly ground black pepper

8 large eggs

3 tablespoons cream cheese, cut up and softened

⅓ cup shredded Gruyère cheese

1. Place the leek in a large bowl and cover with cold water. Swish the leek to remove any grit. Lift the leek out into a colander. Repeat if the leek is very dirty.

2. Heat the oil in a large nonstick skillet over medium heat. Add the leek and cook, stirring occasionally, until tender and golden, about 7 minutes. Stir in a pinch each of salt and pepper.

3. Meanwhile, beat the eggs with the cream cheese and a pinch each of salt and pepper until well blended.

4. Add the egg mixture to the leeks in the skillet. Cook, stirring, until the eggs are almost set but still creamy. Sprinkle with the Gruyère.

Slow Cooker Split Pea Soup

SERVES 8

4 carrots, finely chopped

2 celery stalks, finely chopped

1 large onion, finely chopped

2 garlic cloves, finely chopped

3 fresh thyme sprigs

2 smoked turkey wings

1 pound green split peas, picked over, rinsed, and drained

6 cups lower-sodium chicken or vegetable broth

Salt and freshly ground black pepper

1. Combine the carrots, celery, onion, garlic, thyme, turkey, green split peas, broth, and a pinch each of salt and freshly ground black pepper in the bowl of a 5½-quart slow cooker. Stir until well mixed.

2. Cook on the low setting for 8 hours or on the high setting for 5 hours. It is done when the peas are very tender.

3. Remove and discard the thyme. Remove the turkey wings. If desired, pull off the meat, shred, and return the meat to the soup. Discard the bones. Season to taste with salt and pepper.

Hummus

MAKES 2½ CUPS

2 15-ounce cans chickpeas (garbanzo beans)

⅓ cup fresh lemon juice

⅓ cup tahini (sesame paste)

1 garlic clove, crushed

⅛ teaspoon cayenne pepper, optional

Salt and freshly ground black pepper

¼ cup extra-virgin olive oil

¼ teaspoon sweet paprika, optional

1 tablespoon chopped fresh flat-leaf parsley, optional

1. Pulse the chickpeas, lemon juice, tahini, garlic, cayenne, and a pinch each of salt and pepper in a food processor until almost smooth.

2. With the machine running, add the oil and 2 tablespoons water in a steady stream. Add more water for a thinner consistency if desired. Puree until smooth.

3. Sprinkle with paprika and parsley if desired before serving.

Coriander Butternut Squash Soup

SERVES 4

2 tablespoons butter

1 medium onion, chopped

Salt and freshly ground black pepper

1 teaspoon coriander seeds

1 large (2¾-pound) butternut squash, halved, peeled, seeded, and chopped, or 1 package (20 ounces) fresh precut butternut squash

5 cups canned low-sodium chicken broth or water

¼ cup packed fresh cilantro leaves, chopped, optional

¼ cup sour cream, optional

1. Melt the butter in a large saucepan over medium heat. Add the onion, season with salt and pepper, and cook, stirring occasionally, until tender, about 8 minutes. Add the coriander seeds and cook, stirring, until golden brown and fragrant, about 2 minutes. Add the squash and stir well, then add the broth or water.

2. Bring the mixture to a boil over high heat, then lower the heat to maintain a steady simmer. Cook until the squash is tender enough for a knife to easily pierce through, about 30 minutes.

3. Transfer the soup to a blender and carefully puree until smooth. Work in batches if necessary. Return the soup to the saucepan and season to taste with salt and pepper. Keep warm over low heat if you're not serving immediately.

4. Divide the soup among serving bowls. Top with cilantro and sour cream.

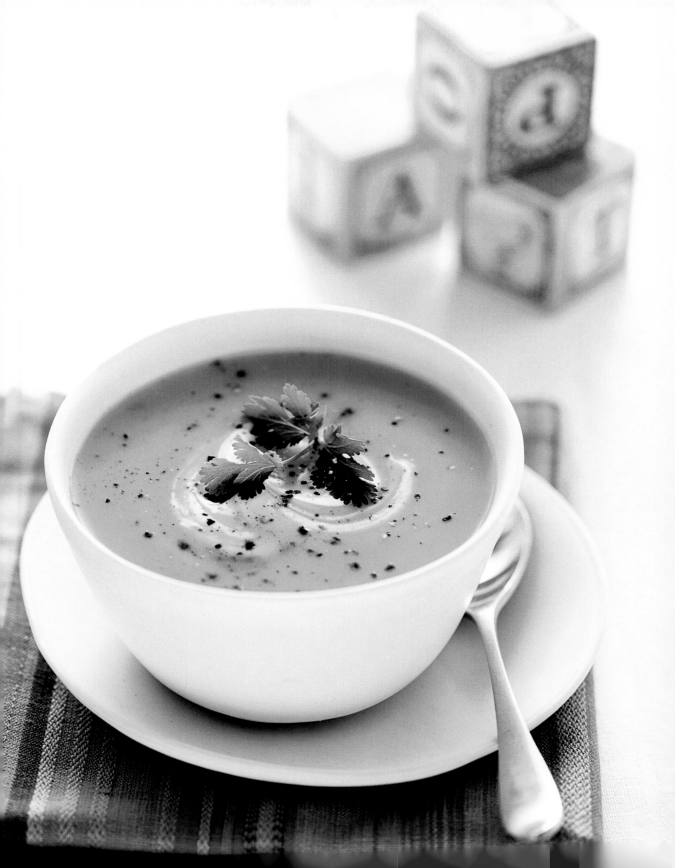

Orange-Braised Baby Carrots

SERVES 4

1 pound baby carrots

¾ cup fresh orange juice

1 tablespoon butter

Salt and freshly ground black pepper

1. Place the carrots, juice, butter, and a pinch each of salt and pepper in a medium saucepan. Bring to a boil over medium heat.

2. Simmer, stirring occasionally, until the carrots are tender and the juice has evaporated to a glaze clinging to the carrots, about 17 minutes.

Celery Root and Potato Puree

SERVES 4

1 pound all-purpose potatoes, peeled and coarsely chopped

1 celery root (celeriac), trimmed, peeled, and coarsely chopped

½ cup reduced-fat (2%) milk, warmed

2 tablespoons butter

Salt and freshly ground black pepper

1. Place the potatoes and celery root in a large saucepan and cover with cold water. Bring to a boil over high heat, then reduce the heat to medium-low and simmer until tender, about 15 minutes.

2. Drain and transfer to a food processor, along with the milk, butter, and a pinch each of salt and pepper. Puree just until smooth. You can also transfer the potatoes and celery root to a large bowl and mash with the milk, butter, and a pinch each of salt and pepper.

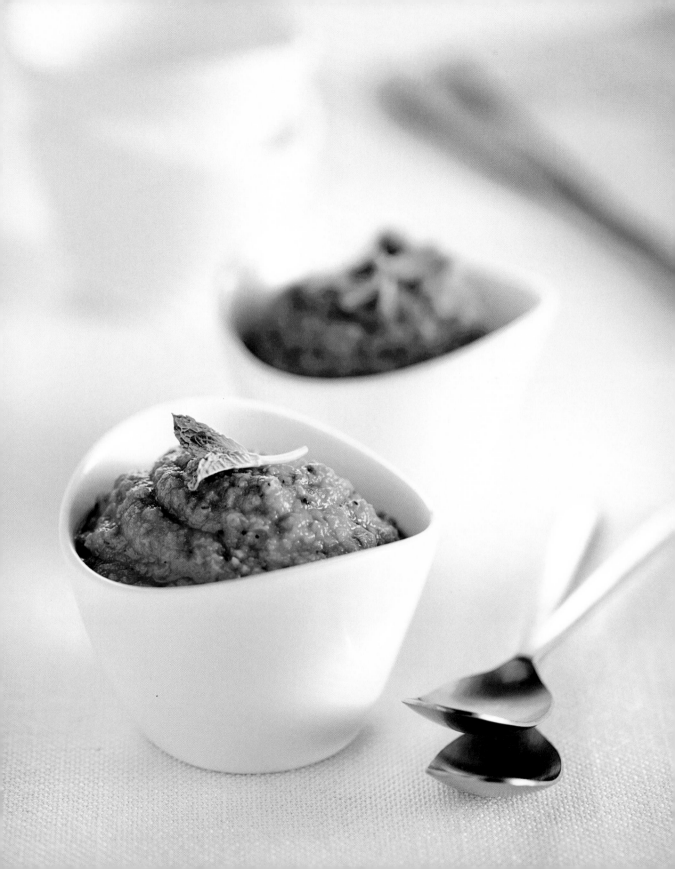

Minted Pea Puree

SERVES 4

1 pound frozen peas

½ cup packed fresh mint leaves

2 tablespoons whole milk

2 tablespoons butter

Salt and freshly ground black pepper

1. Combine the peas, mint, and ¼ cup water in a large saucepan. Bring the mixture to a boil over high heat. Cover, reduce the heat to medium, and cook, stirring occasionally, until the peas are bright green and tender, about 7 minutes.

2. Drain the mixture, then transfer to a food processor. Add the milk and butter and puree until smooth. Season to taste with salt and pepper.

Homemade Apple-Pear Sauce

MAKES ABOUT 2½ CUPS

2 organic Golden Delicious apples, cored and cut into 8 wedges

2 organic Bartlett pears, cored and cut into 8 wedges

1. In a saucepan fitted with a steamer insert or basket, bring 1 inch of water to a boil.

2. Add the apples and pears to the steamer, cover, and cook until very tender, about 15 minutes.

3. Transfer the apples and pears to a blender, along with ½ cup of the cooking water. Blend, adding more water for a thinner consistency if desired, until pureed to desired consistency.

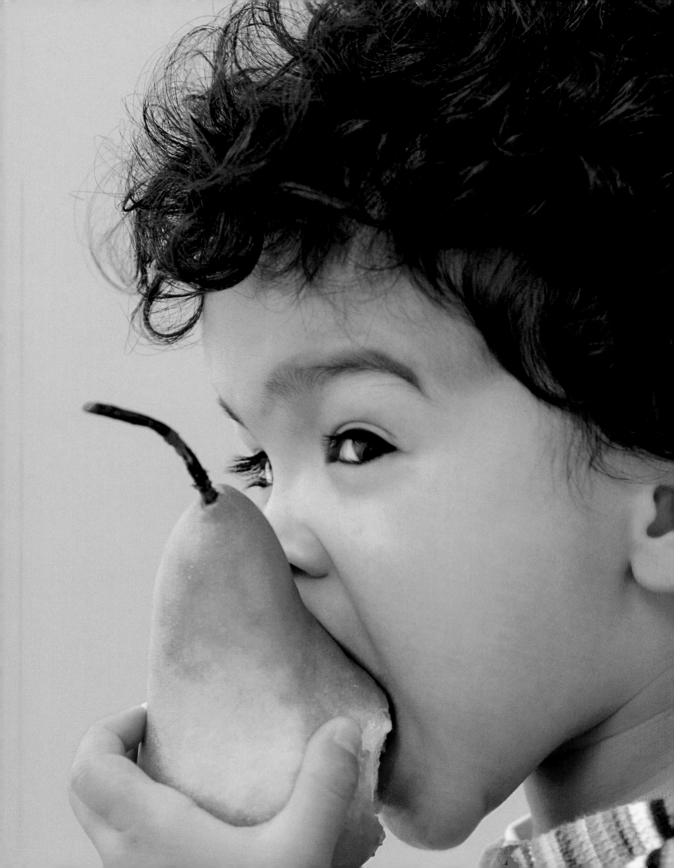

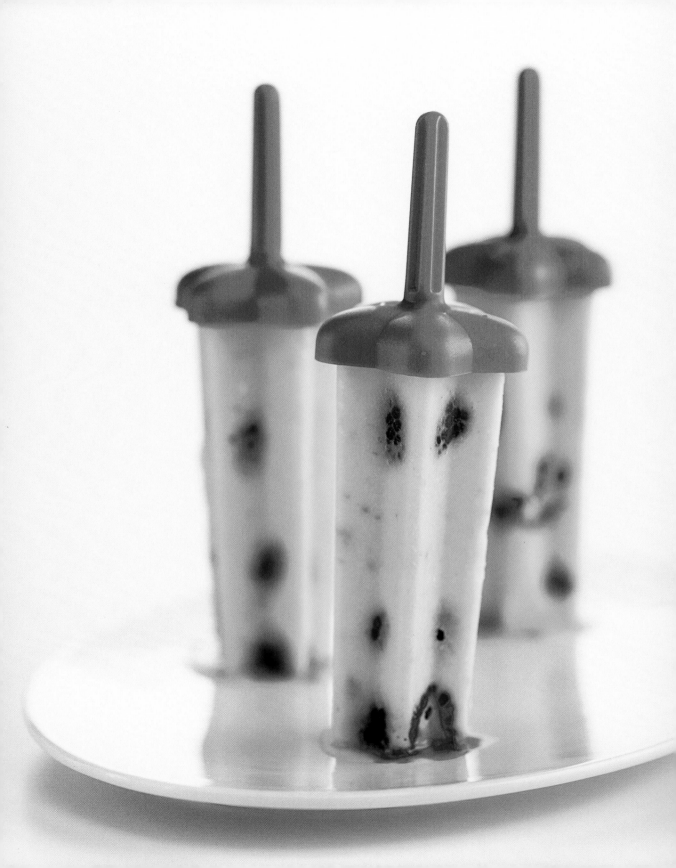

Peach Pops

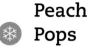

MAKES 8 POPS

½ pint raspberries

½ cup plus 1 tablespoon sugar, preferably superfine

1 pound ripe peaches, pitted and chopped

1 cup plain whole-milk yogurt

1 teaspoon fresh lemon juice

1. Combine the raspberries and 1 tablespoon sugar in a small bowl. Let stand.

2. Combine the peaches, yogurt, lemon juice, and remaining ½ cup sugar in a blender. Puree until very smooth. Add the raspberries and gently fold in with a rubber spatula until just swirled in.

3. Divide the mixture among 8 pop molds. Freeze and insert pop sticks according to the package's directions.

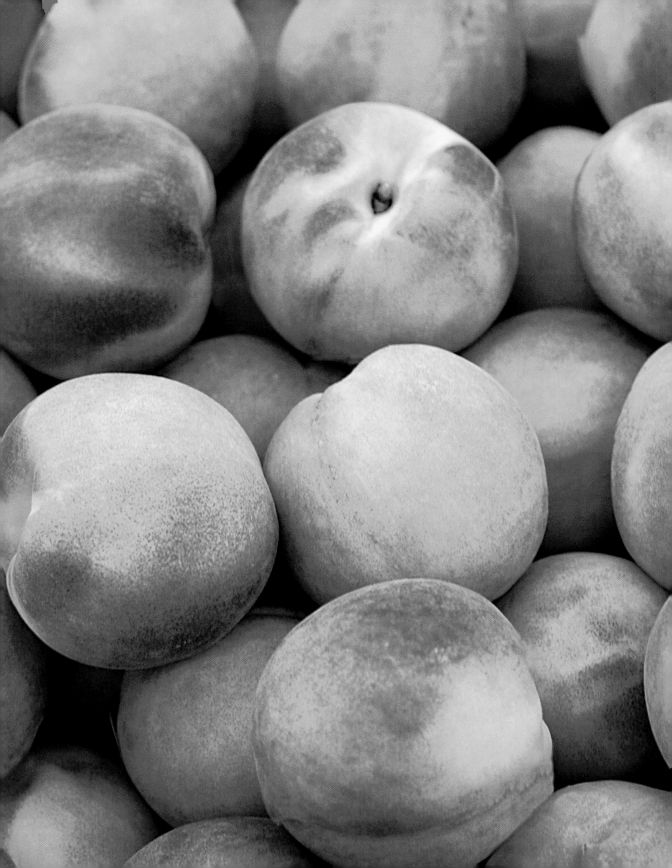

Chapter 5

At the Table Together

FROM 12 TO 18 MONTHS AND BEYOND

As you look at your healthy nursling—on the brink of walking, talking toddlerhood!—it's amazing to think that one short year ago he was such a tiny little bundle of mystery. You have journeyed a long way together in a very short time, and there is so much more to look forward to. Breastfeeding, even as it occurs with less frequency than it did in those early months, remains a precious and special way of connecting throughout the day, particularly as your child develops a healthy independence and curiosity about the world around him.

As he enters his second year of life, he is a regular and lively presence in the kitchen, keeping the cooks company, and at the table, where he observes and participates in his own way. Perhaps he is demanding tastes of everything, or maybe he's still getting a feel for solids. He may be waving a spoon and grabbing for everyone's cup; he may prefer his fingers over any other utensils. Continue to let him lead the way as he progresses toward more solid foods. Though he may be less dependent on your milk as a primary food source as he moves (crawls, walks, then runs!) into toddlerhood and beyond, he is still entirely dependent upon you for wholesome and healthy meals and snacks, and will be for quite some time.

Now more than ever, the food you keep in your home is especially important to your child's health and that of your whole family. What you choose to purchase, prepare, and serve will probably be showing up on his plate in some form. Just as important, he is watching and taking his cues from you, his first teacher in life. If you model good eating habits, you're increasing his chances for making good choices, too.

It's a long way off, but someday he will be a hungry boy standing in a school lunch line . . . a hungry teenager hanging out after school at a friend's house . . . a hungry young adult with his first stove and a refrigerator to fill. Will he go for the cheeseburger or the turkey wrap? The candy or the fruit? Will he know how to put together a simple breakfast or will he skip it or hit a drive-through? At the grocery store, will he spend his money on microwave burritos or the ingredients for a simple but satisfying meal?

As you snuggle with your healthy, well-fed nursling, it's practically impossible to imagine that someday he will have such choices to make—choices that will impact his health for life. By choosing breastfeeding, you've given him an excellent nutritional foundation. By choosing to eat healthfully and setting an example that he can follow, you're extending that beneficial foundation beyond childhood and into adulthood.

Your Nutritional Needs: Now and Looking Ahead

You may be months or years away from weaning your child, though we'd like to point out that "weaning" has more than one definition. For some cultures, the moment a baby takes any nourishment in addition to mother's milk, be it formula or solids, that is weaning. For others, weaning means the total cessation of breastfeeding. In **The Womanly Art of Breastfeeding**, we point out that actually it's a bit of both: as soon as your nursling has any food or drink other than breast milk, the weaning process has begun. It does not end until your child breastfeeds for the last time. How long does weaning last? It can take days or years. Ideally, the breastfeeding relationship will continue until your baby outgrows the need. Above all, it's a personal choice that only you and your child can make.

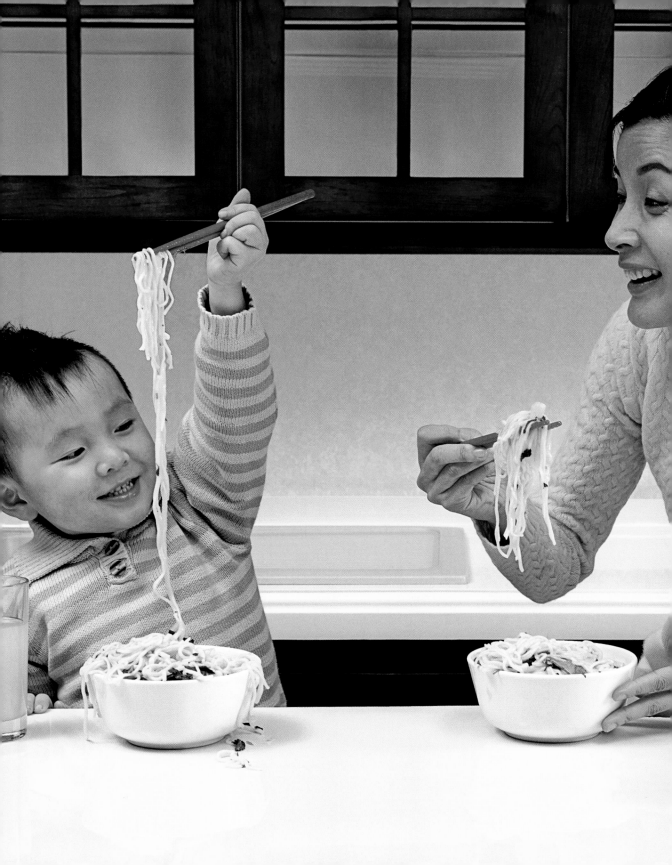

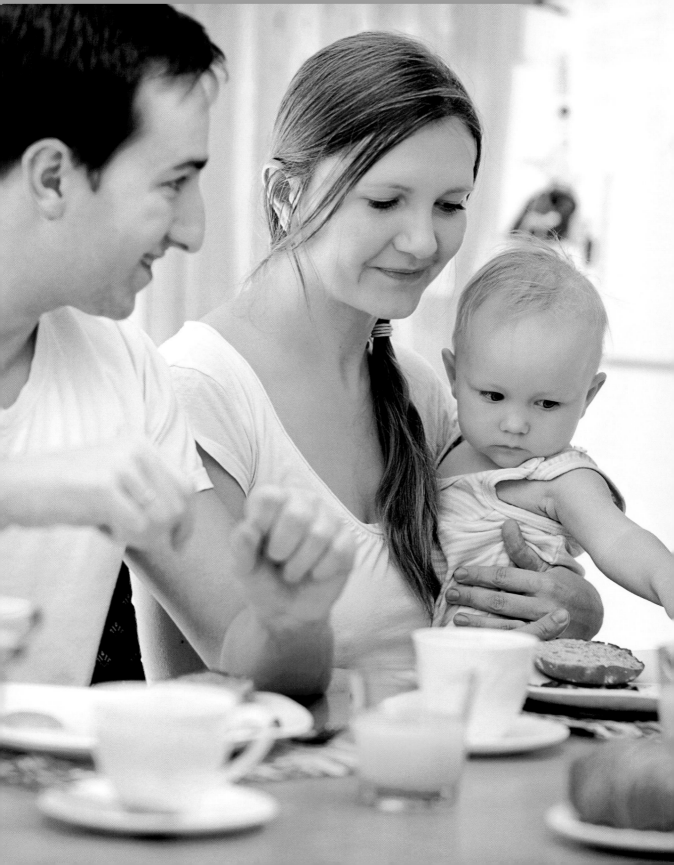

No matter where you are on your motherhood journey, you may be wondering about your own nutritional needs once the weaning process begins. As you know, mothers generally take in extra calories to support maternal and fetal health throughout pregnancy, as well as additional calories when breastfeeding begins; as we pointed out in the last chapter, at 6 months a breastfeeding mother needs yet another small increase in calories because by that time she has depleted her maternal fat stores (see page 152). There comes a time when extra calories are no longer needed by a breastfeeding mother, but it depends in part on when the weaning process begins and the rate at which it progresses.

One simple and natural way to evaluate your calorie needs is to consider your postpartum weight loss. Are you heading in the direction you'd like to be moving in? Have you hit your goal? For some women, the old "9 months up, 9 months down" adage is fairly reliable. For others it's just that—an old adage. If you are holding on to extra pregnancy weight gain that you'd like to shed and get to a suitable BMI (see page 5), you can begin to pull back on those additional calories you added. Talk to your health care provider about a safe level of weight loss, if that is your goal—usually no more than a pound a week.

Continue to strive for balanced levels of lean protein, complex carbohydrates, and plenty of fruits and vegetables as you put together your daily meals, adding dairy or another source of calcium. You still need 1,000 milligrams of calcium daily for bone health (including teeth). Maternal bone loss during lactation is approximately 3 to 7 percent, but this is rapidly regained after weaning. If you plan to get pregnant again, folate remains a vital nutrient for fetal brain development, and you may want to take in more than the recommended 400 micrograms per day (see page 60). Otherwise, a varied and healthy diet is the only "diet" you need—for life.

Exercise (Or, Another Reason Children Make Your Heart Beat a Little Faster)

While regular exercising may feel easier on your body now that you have your energy back, it may be harder in one regard: finding the time. (Ask

Exercise (Or, Another Reason Children Make Your Heart Beat a Little Faster) (CONTINUED)

anyone, though—this seems to be true whether you're a mom or not! See pages 119–20 for more on exercise.) The good news is that by now, it's truly possible to bring your baby along for the ride—literally.

By 1 year of age, most babies can ride safely in a rear-mounted bike seat or be pulled in a bike trailer; according to the AAP, a child should be able to sit well unsupported and should have the neck strength to support the wearing of a lightweight helmet. If biking isn't your thing, a sturdy "baby jogger" stroller will get you and your child out and about. (Even with a jogger, a lightweight helmet is recommended for baby. Also, if you obtain used bike equipment or a jogging stroller, have it looked over as a safety precaution and tuned up if necessary by a bike mechanic before you take baby for a spin.) If jogging or running isn't your thing, walk, walk, walk. If the weather is right, get your partner out for a stroll after dinner and do some family moves after family meals.

No matter how or where you choose to get your exercise, if you're physically active—and, even better, if you can include your child in your exercise routine—you're modeling a healthy lifestyle and setting a great example for her to follow. Plus it's just fun.

"Boy, is it hard to get started. The first week or two of adding exercise to your overtired body is sort of excruciating. But it gets oh so much better, and your body and mind will love you for it!"

From Baby to Big Kid: Keeping Up with Your Child's Nutrition

Mothers nourish—with their milk, then with food and drink, and always with love. No matter how we feed our children, we mothers also tend to worry when our children don't eat the way we think they should.

Our worrying starts when they are tiny babies. Before we allow ourselves to settle into a successful breastfeeding relationship, we may be made to fret over whether or

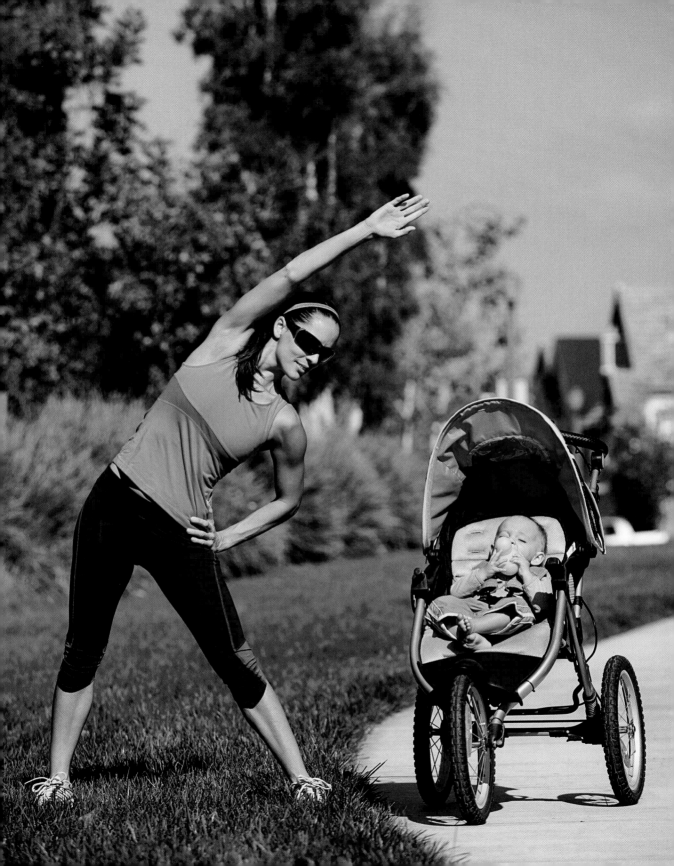

not they're getting enough milk. When they begin solids, it can start anew if we question whether or not they're eating enough, or if they are eating the right things. The worrying may kick in again when they start preschool or kindergarten and we aren't present at lunchtime or for snacks. As they grow, our concerns may be about not enough veggies or calcium, too much sugar or fat, or what (and how) they are eating when we're not with them.

Early on, we pointed out that we think there is already too much worry and guilt surrounding eating. When that free-floating food anxiety collides with the emotional powerhouse of motherhood, everyone—parents and kids—can lose their appetite! **She's not eating any green vegetables. . . . She won't eat what I cooked. . . . I think she's sneaking candy and soda!**

It's time to step back and stop worrying. We are not trying to ignore the fact that some children can and will develop health issues ranging from food allergies and nutritional deficiencies to weight-related problems. We're also not trying to deny the reality that at a certain point your child will make her own decisions about food and they may not be ones you'll approve of. However, for right now, you are doing the best thing possible—breastfeeding—to protect your child's health through good nutrition. Looking ahead, you'll continue to do the best thing—feeding your child wholesome food, keeping it in your kitchen and serving it for breakfast, lunch, and dinner, and giving her an appetite for the same "good stuff" that will keep you healthy.

Depending on your child's age and how much solid food she is getting now, her nutritional needs will vary, so you may wish to check in with your health care provider for age-appropriate recommendations on protein, calcium, iron, and other important dietary components. However, here are a few facts to replace the worries with regard to how most children eat.

1. **They don't eat a lot because their stomachs are really small.** Little tummies fill up quickly, so children stop eating when they are full. Don't push food if your child doesn't want it—learning to feel full is extremely important, as that is the mechanism that stops us from overeating. Let your child learn to follow his own appetite cues, eating when he's hungry and stopping when he is full. Serve small amounts and let him ask for more.

Prepare healthy snacks to offer between meals when hunger strikes—and it will!

2. **Just because they refuse it today doesn't mean they'll refuse it forever.** Children are open to trying new foods and new tastes—they aren't born hating cauliflower. But they can also be cautious and stubborn (these are survival skills, after all). Just because he won't try peas today doesn't mean he'll never eat them. He may just want the butternut squash for now. Offer the new food again another day—there will be plenty of opportunities. Another reason your baby may balk at a new food: a breastfed baby is exposed to a variety of tastes through his mother's milk, but when he eats a food in its solid form he is probably getting a more concentrated flavor. Give him a chance to get used to it.

3. **Think week, not day.** Monday: two bites of apple. Tuesday: four nibbles of chicken. Wednesday: two servings of green beans. Thursday: a slice of cheese. Friday: nothing. Saturday: scrambled eggs, banana, macaroni and cheese, pear, avocado . . . If you're trying to determine whether your child is eating a balanced diet, nutritionists and other experts suggest it's better to look at a week's worth of food, rather than what he eats in a 24-hour period. Toddlers, especially, are notorious for their "grazing" style of eating. As they mature, their diets will become more consistent. (For now, he's experimenting with holding a cracker in his mouth for a couple of hours.)

4. **Don't fret about fat.** Because we're constantly told to watch our fat intake, many parents worry unnecessarily over limiting fat in the diets of babies and toddlers, but for most healthy children this is not necessary (and restricting it too stringently could be dangerous). For brain development and growth young children **need healthy fats** from whole foods (not trans and saturated fats from processed foods or greasy fried foods). Lowering fat intake becomes more important as they near preschool—but it's a nonissue for the typical baby or toddler who is growing properly.

5. **Sometimes a green bean is just a green bean.** Food can become an emotional issue for many of us. We want our children to eat properly (and not rub food in their hair), and we grow concerned when they don't do as

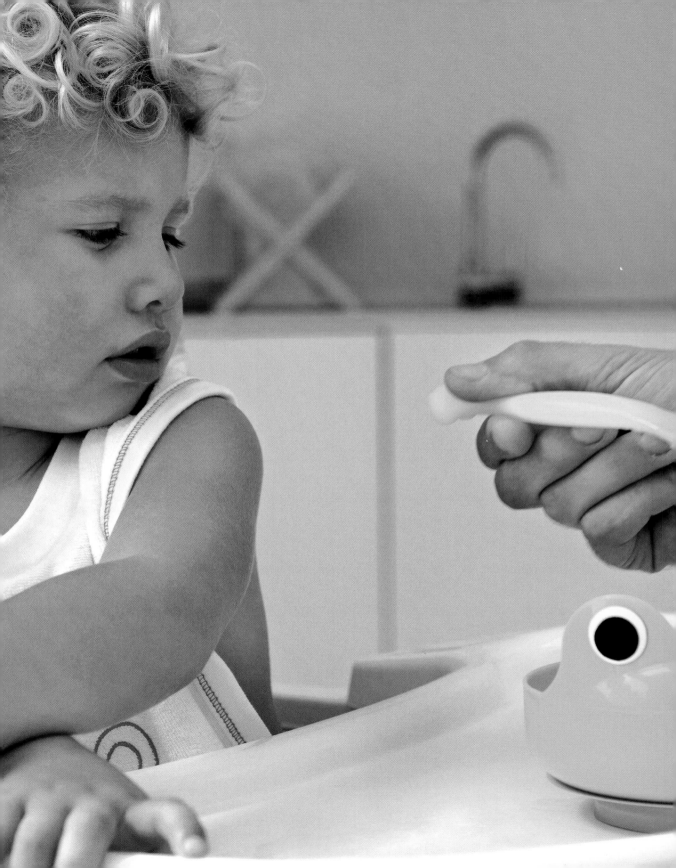

we desire. If they reject what we prepare, it only means they are rejecting a food they don't want at that particular moment—not the healthy lifestyle lesson we're hoping to imprint upon them. From the start, it's crucial to create a calm, positive feeding environment where a child can confidently follow his appetite cues, even if things get messy and some foods go uneaten. Solid food is a brand-new world. As with all the new worlds he will discover as he grows, guide your child through it and keep him safe, but give him some freedom to explore and learn.

"At 21 months, Joe **can** use a spoon correctly if he feels like it, but often he doesn't. He hates being spoon-fed, so I stopped that ages ago. If he wants to eat yogurt with his face, okay. I prefer it when he uses a spoon, but that's not that neat, either."

—SARAH

"At about 10 months both my sons could eat a bowl of yogurt or applesauce very well with a spoon. I always put a spoon on their tray right from the beginning and they eventually picked it up and used it. One could eat an entire meal with a spoon or fork very well before he was 1. The other still tends to hold the spoon in one hand and shove food in his mouth with his free hand."

—KELLI

The Family Meal—for Baby, Too

As the months go by, you'll want to offer the same healthy foods that you and the rest of your family are eating, but you'll also want to be confident that your baby can safely chew and swallow new and more complex textures. In the last chapter you read about the stages of sucking, chewing, and swallowing that allow a baby to manage solids as she nears the end of her first year of life, and we offered some ideas for appropriate first foods. By 12 months, she can chew and swallow mixed (soft and slightly hard) textures. Eventually she'll be able to handle harder textures such as most crackers or thin pretzels. At around 18 months, a baby can manage harder foods that require grinding—for example, raw vegetables, raw and dried fruits, and firmer-textured meats (such as steak).

At a certain point, there is very little a baby with growing teeth and stronger jaws **can't** chew and swallow (including, unfortunately, many items that are not food)—all the more reason why you can comfortably make one meal for your family. Still, be aware that some foods, such as too-large pieces of meat or hard vegetables, can cause choking even among older children; make sure your baby and any young children are supervised when eating. Even some healthy snack foods, such as grapes, nuts, and plain popcorn, are choking hazards for babies and youngsters.

It needn't be seasoned or served the same way, but try to get into the habit of making your baby's food from the ingredients of your family meal. You'll save yourself time and money—no need to buy prepared baby food (see below)—and you'll avoid the fate of making more than one meal. Talk to any mother who has morphed into a short-order cook ("I make chicken for Susan, pasta for Mark, and fish for my husband and me") and chances are she'll tell you that it all started when her kids began eating solids! (See the next section for stopping picky eating before it takes hold.)

 ## (Baby) Food for Thought: Should You Buy the Jar?

If you are pressed for time or your schedule keeps you out of the kitchen most of the day, you may be tempted to purchase prepared baby food to save time and work. Certainly the selection now is better than it once was. Beyond the jar, you'll find plenty of organic products, including premium brands of frozen baby food. (In some cities you can even have fresh baby food delivered to your door.) But regardless of how much you pay, is it any good? If you reach for the jar (or the frozen food cubes in the fancy box), keep in mind the following.

Pure vegetables or fruit are usually okay, but many commercial jarred baby foods have added water or starchy fillers. You can probably offer a soft-textured fruit such as banana, thinned if necessary with breast milk. That's a much better nutritional deal for baby than a jar of "peach-banana medley," which contains peaches, bananas, water, and modified tapioca starch for thickener (plus other additives and preservatives). Also, why not give your child the honest flavor of a single fruit or vegetable, as opposed to a flavor mash-up, particularly if she's trying new foods for the first time?

If you buy a baby food product featuring meat mixed with vegetables or pasta, consider this: When we feed babies meat or chicken, we are doing it to provide them with protein and iron. Once a food manufacturer adds an ingredient such as pasta or a starchy vegetable (even if it's organically grown), some of the protein and iron content is replaced with carbohydrate. As with fruits and vegetables, poultry, meat, or fish in their purest forms—cooked without additives and fillers—offer the most nutritional benefit.

Finally, keep in mind that jarred, pureed baby foods are inconsistent with the baby-led approach to weaning, which we recommend. Rather than give a baby table foods that are pureed and spoon-fed, baby-led weaning involves allowing a baby the freedom to feed himself and set the pace, with appropriate foods in sizes and shapes that he can handle.

If you choose prepared baby food, always select products that are as pure and as close to the original food as possible—read the labels carefully and consider that food manufacturers almost always have to add ingredients you wouldn't use, to thicken their products, give them a long shelf life, and make them look more attractive. It probably takes just as long to read through all those ingredients as it does to take some peas off your own plate and shred a few pieces of the same chicken you're having. For more on preparing your own food for baby, and on baby and toddler nutrition, we suggest **Whole Foods for Babies and Toddlers** by Margaret Kenda, published by La Leche League International.[1]

What About Snacks and Treats?

As we said earlier, small stomachs fill up quickly, but they don't stay full for long. Active toddlers and preschoolers need healthy snacks between meals. They aren't usually eating large portions at breakfast, lunch, and dinner, and these small folks are on the go, so they are bound to get hungry. There is no shortage of kid-size prepared snack foods in most supermarkets—100-calorie "snack packs" are all the rage, and miniature juice boxes with cartoon characters are hard to avoid. (For more on kids and juice, see page 211–12.)

The problem is many of these child-size portions and snack foods are full of the stuff you don't want your child to snack on—sugar, sodium, empty calories. (And 100 calories for a snack is actually a lot for a little body.) If this is your first child, you have yet to encounter the world of preschool snacks, after-school snacks, soccer game team snacks, morning snacks to bring to school, and every other configuration of children and snacks. Take the time now to unravel the answer to what makes a healthy snack for a young eater (hint: it almost always comes out of your own kitchen, not a bag or a box).

Remember when you were trying to put together your own healthy snacks when you were pregnant and, later, when you were beginning with breastfeeding? You quickly learned to take a pass on the prepared snack foods and put together your own supply of hunger-busters. It's time to do the same for your child. Many of the same whole, unprocessed foods you turned to can be served to your child, though of course consider her age and her ability to chew and swallow. (Avoid any food that could be a choking hazard.) Look back at the snack ideas in Chapters 1 and 2 and you'll find plenty of inspiration.

Toddlers and preschoolers like interesting shapes and colors, and as they get more dexterous, they like to dip and dunk and mix their foods. Try red and green apple slices and offer plain or vanilla yogurt as a dip, or hummus (see page 183) and crackers or veggies. If you're on the go, bring along cut-up fruit (or an orange or banana you can peel on the spot), turkey slices, hard-boiled eggs, cheese and crackers, or a homemade oatmeal cookie (see page 100) or muffin.

So what if you are on the go and away from home with your suddenly hun-

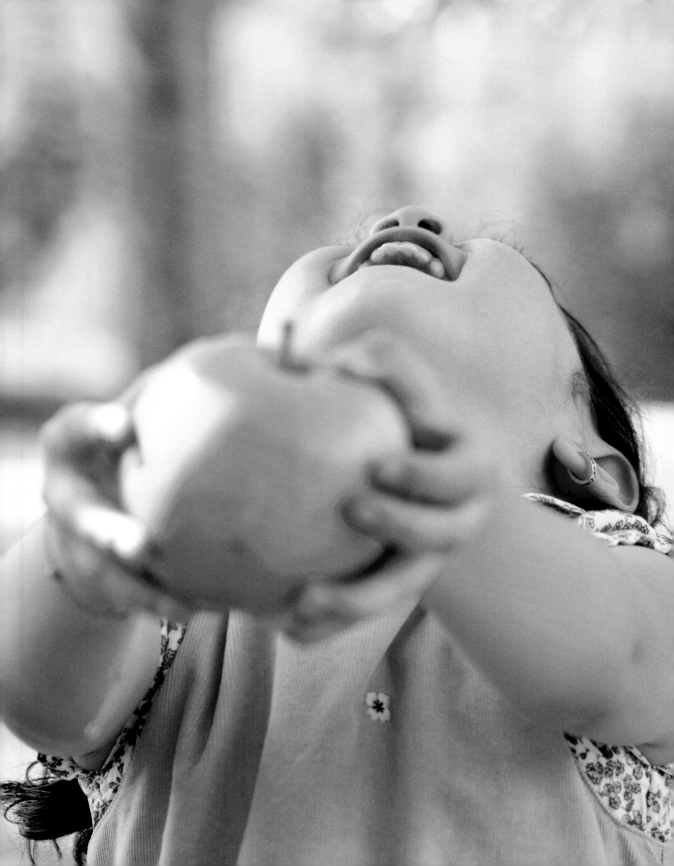

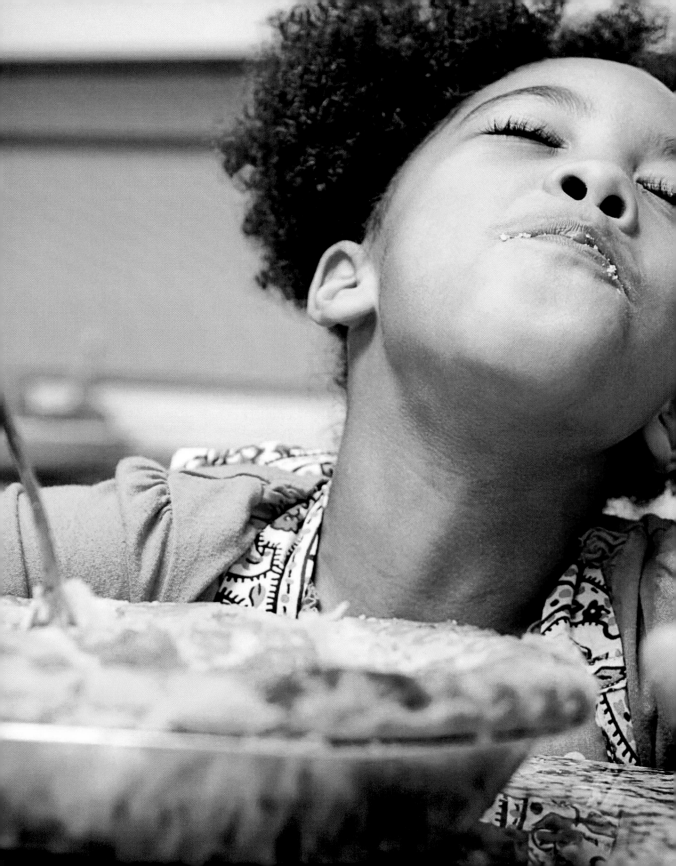

gry child and you are snackless? There isn't a banana in sight. Should you buy the package of chocolate-covered peanuts, the pretzels, or the granola bar? How about that 100-calorie bag of animal crackers? Consider the fat, sugar, and sodium content, and remember as well the 15/5 rule (see page 25)—it works for children, too.

At a certain point, you may look down at your child's snack and discover that it is, in fact, a treat—a cupcake, an ice pop, a piece of chocolate. Even if you are a stickler for what your child consumes, treats happen (you may not be there when his cake-baking great-grandma lets him lick the icing off the spoon). It's okay. Just label these foods as the treats they truly are, and never as everyday snacks. Teach your child the difference between healthy, wholesome snack foods and special-occasion treats. As one mom likes to repeat to her kids, "A treat is a treat, a snack is a snack"—simple but true. In a few years' time, when your child is old enough, teach her how to put together her own healthy snacks and make sure your kitchen and refrigerator are filled with good options. Most of all, try to set an example yourself when you choose your own snacks and treats, and encourage your partner to do so as well.

Finally, don't use a sugary snack as a reward. **If you're a good girl while we're shopping, you can have a cookie when we get home. . . . If you stop crying, you can have an ice cream cone. . . . You get a cupcake for being so nice to your little brother.** This just teaches us that we can congratulate ourselves with sugar for getting through tough times—even into adulthood. There is nothing wrong with a sweet treat from time to time, but don't give power to the sweet stuff.

Kids and Juice

The ubiquitous juice box did not exist a generation ago, but now it has its own considerable section in the grocery store and gets packed into lunchboxes, tucked into the tote bag or stroller, and handed out with a child-size snack millions of times a day. If it's 100 percent fruit juice—not a "juice drink" or "carbonated juice beverage"—is it bad for your child?

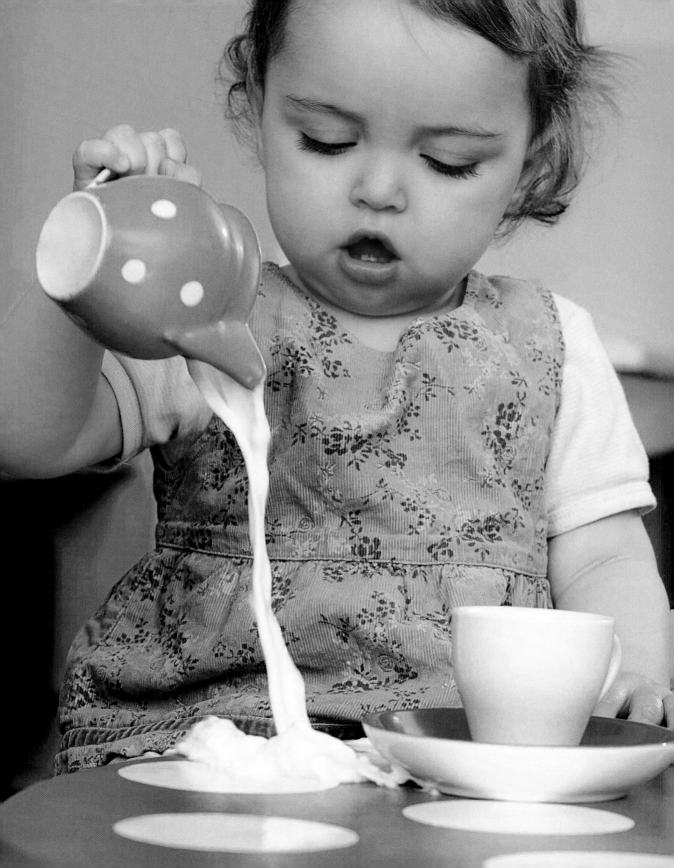

Kids and Juice (CONTINUED)

The short answer is no—if it's pure juice with no sugar added and consumed in moderation (see guidelines below). But many children drink too much juice, and it has a lot of sugar; even a 4-ounce mini-box of pure orange or apple juice has about 2½ teaspoons of sugar. It's natural fruit sugar (fructose), but it's still sugar, and it contributes to a child's daily calorie intake.

Children have small stomachs, and if they fill up on juice, they may not have room for more nutritious drinks and foods. Babies generally like the sweet taste of juice, but milk—breast milk if they are still nursing—is a healthier drink, or water may quench their thirst adequately. For thirsty older children, offer water first, and discourage them from meeting their needs for fluids with sweet, high-calorie juice. It could encourage a taste for sweet beverages later on—including soda.

Limit a child's daily juice intake as follows:[2]

- For ages 6 to 12 months, no more than 4 ounces
- For toddlers and preschoolers, no more than 6 ounces
- For school-age children, no more than 8 ounces

If possible, make your own juice from fresh fruits, and dilute pure juice with plain water (or seltzer, for older kids who are ready for some fizz). Better yet, offer fiber-containing, juicy fresh fruit and water.

Putting It All Together: The Family Meal

Not long ago, a mom we know was grocery shopping when she observed two grandmotherly women of a certain age greeting each other fondly, exchanging pleasantries about their adult children and grandchildren, their retired spouses and active lives, and their mutual acquaintances. "Well," said one as she prepared to head off, "have a great day!" "Ugh," the other huffed, gripping her

"If I'm cooking dinner and my husband is playing with the baby, when the baby gets hungry I take the baby to nurse and will give my husband a summary of what's going on for dinner: 'That timer is for the chicken, the other timer is for the potatoes, and I was planning on steaming some green beans. . . . ' My husband then takes over cooking dinner and getting it on the table. During dinner we take turns with the baby so we both have a chance to eat. After dinner is playtime, then bedtime routines for our toddler and baby. We continue to trade off until both kids are asleep. After the kids are asleep we both take turns doing cleanup from dinner and making the toddler's lunch for preschool the next day. Often we'll start some prep for the next night's dinner."

shopping cart and rolling her eyes at the produce, "I would, if only I didn't have to make dinner . . . **again**!"

For this woman, being in charge of the family meal hadn't ended when her children left home—perhaps because her spouse still looked to her and her alone for getting food on the table. (This anecdote is a great argument for making sure that your partner, and your children when they are old enough, are self-sufficient in the kitchen and the grocery store!) The fact remains that in many households, even in a time when dads and partners pitch in more with housework and child care than in previous generations, it is often moms who take on much of the domestic burden, particularly if they don't work outside the home.

Embracing a "share the care" approach to family life usually benefits both partners in a relationship; housework, cooking, bill paying, errands, and the like get done faster when two adults tackle the to-do list 50/50-style, freeing up more time for both parents to be involved with kids. It's easier to establish this equal footing with your partner if you do it when your children are young. As a nursing mother, you'll find that it's challenging—but certainly not impossible—to share with your partner the responsibility of feeding your child. (In **The Womanly Art of Breastfeeding**, we offer many suggestions for part-

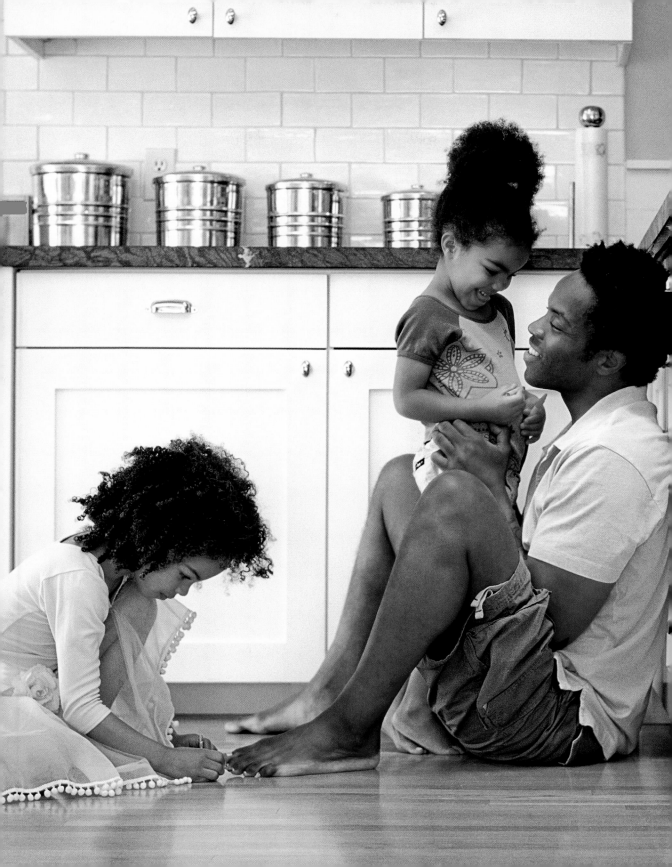

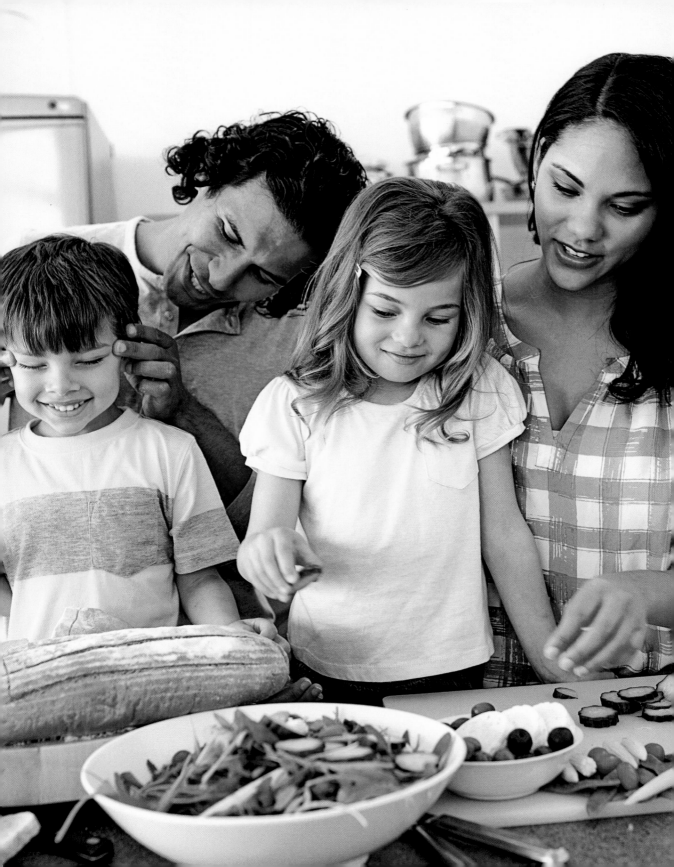

ner involvement in nursling care that do not involve bottle-feeding, from baby wearing to acting as a protective buffer between you and those who may not support breastfeeding.)

However, even before solids enter the picture, your partner can play a major role at mealtime, whether it's prepping ingredients, doing the actual cooking, helping to feed the smallest eater at the table, or fielding the chunks of canta-loupe that are being tossed merrily from your baby's chair.

Throughout your pregnancy and then after your baby was born, we encour-aged you to accept offers of help (and food), including assistance from your partner. Don't stop now, as the journey is just beginning, and feeding your fam-ily involves more than simply planning a menu and buying groceries.

If you are a single mom, perhaps you have older kids who can pitch in at mealtime. Maybe you put together a support network of friends and family who came through for you when your baby was new to the world; now that your child is moving beyond babyhood, let them know they are still needed and appreciated—and would they like to come over for dinner?

Whatever your source of support, whomever you consider family, the first step in putting together the family meal is to make it a family effort!

⚡ Make-Ahead Recipes

- Black Bean Salsa, page 144

- Hummus, page 183

- Soy-Lime Marinated Salmon, page 133

- Slow Cooker Split Pea Soup, page 182

- Dandy Candy, page 241

- Slow Cooker Chuck Roast with Carrots, Tomatoes, and Potatoes, page 177

- Avocado Salsa, page 143

- Quinoa Pilaf with White Beans, Feta Cheese, and Summer Vegetables, page 139

- Savory Baked French Toast, page 138

Make-Ahead Recipes (CONTINUED)

- Slow Cooker Vegetarian Chili, page 136

- La Leche League Baking Mix, page 97

- Easy Microwave Eggplant Dip for Crudités, page 95

- Minestrone with White Beans and Loads of Vegetables, page 85

- Slow Cooker Spinach Lasagna, page 84

- Calico Bean Salad, page 54

- Tabbouleh (Bulgur and Lentil Salad), page 49

Feeding Yourself, Feeding Your Family: It's All Connected Now

If you are a first-time mother, you've gone from eating alone or with your partner to having a constant companion with you at mealtime. Even if this is not your first child, a major change has occurred at the table. You've added a new place for a new eater, one who is here to stay for a good long while.

He may not eat a lot to start, but at some point four pieces of pasta eaten with his little fingers will turn into a plate of dexterously-twisted-onto-his-fork spaghetti and meatballs and a side of broccoli (and you will hear, "Mom, can I have seconds?"). Remember when you had a newborn and everyone would tell you, "Sleep when the baby sleeps"? It's time to adapt that model for food. We're not saying, "Eat what the baby eats," but we are saying, "Let your baby eat what you eat." In other words, as we said above, aim to cook one meal and feed everyone. Here are some reasons to do so:

Everyone—not just the children—eats well. By now, we hope we've given you enough reasons (and recipes) for choosing to eat whole, unprocessed foods. From the moment you became pregnant, your nutrition and your child's became entwined. Now the relationship continues, between you and a growing family. Through breastfeeding, you reduced the risk factors for health problems ranging from allergies to obesity. Through healthy home-cooked meals, you can continue to contribute to your child's health—and you'll eat better, too. Keep the good food around and you'll never be unprepared for a hungry child (or adult, including you).

You'll nip picky eating in the taste buds. Your baby isn't old enough to say, "Yuck, what's that?" when you put a plate in front of her, but unfortunately, that has been known to happen as a child gets older. You can reduce the risk of raising a picky eater if you serve her what you're having (or some version of it, depending on her age) from the very beginning, and introduce her to the tastes that you and your family share. As we have pointed out, breastfed babies naturally eat what their mothers eat, well before they have table food. If you're eating a healthy diet, why do it differently now?

Should you have older children who have managed to stray into picky eating territory, it's not too late to bring them back to the table. First, though, make sure your picky eater isn't the child of a picky parent (including your partner). If she sees the adults around her avoiding vegetables while she is expected to eat hers, or if soda is never allowed but a parent seems to have one in hand at all times, consider the mixed message she is getting. When you eat your green beans, she's more likely to eat hers, too. Remember that children may hesitate to try new foods and that all you can do is keep offering (don't give up) and be patient. Create a happy and warm atmosphere around food; when it becomes tinged with punishments, bribes, and rewards, it doesn't taste very good.

You're preparing your child for tomorrow. Research shows that children who eat a regular family meal (be it breakfast, lunch, or dinner) grow up to have fewer problems with substance abuse, talk to their parents more, and choose healthier diets as adults. Your baby may not be much of a dinner table conversationalist yet, but when she sits down for a meal with her parents, she is entering into a comfortable, trust-filled environment where she can open up to you—now and for years to come. When you share good food with your children and welcome them to the table, you're nourishing them emotionally, too.

The food we grow up with as children can have a powerful hold on us into adulthood. Perhaps it's the grilled cheese sandwich and bowl of tomato soup we remember our own mother serving us for lunch. Maybe it's a traditional dish that reflects our family's ethnicity, a much-loved recipe handed down for generations. It could be as simple as a slice of ice-cold watermelon on a hot day, its sweet refreshment reminding us of family gatherings from summers gone by. (Some of the LLLI Member's Favorite recipes in these pages have been included here precisely because they were favorite flavors for generations of families.)

Admittedly, not all the food we recall from our youth will fit with a healthy way of eating and feeding our families. The fragrant smell of fried bacon and eggs that woke us up each morning . . . the potato chips, root beer, and hot dogs wolfed down at the family picnic table . . . the melting butter and rich sour cream on a perfect baked potato at dinnertime—all remembered fondly, but not the daily diet we strive for now. Today we are armed with knowledge about what goes into our food and its impact on our long-term health. We serve these special foods from time to time, but our everyday meals and snacks are healthier fare.

Your children, like you, will remember the food of their childhood. Your child's first food was your milk—natural, pure, and totally nourishing. As she grows, you can extend this excellent nourishment by offering healthy foods. Perhaps your eating habits improved during pregnancy and when you began breastfeeding, or maybe you were already consuming a good, balanced diet and didn't need to make major adjustments. Either way, it's our hope that you'll continue with confidence down this healthful, whole-foods path.

Bring your family with you.

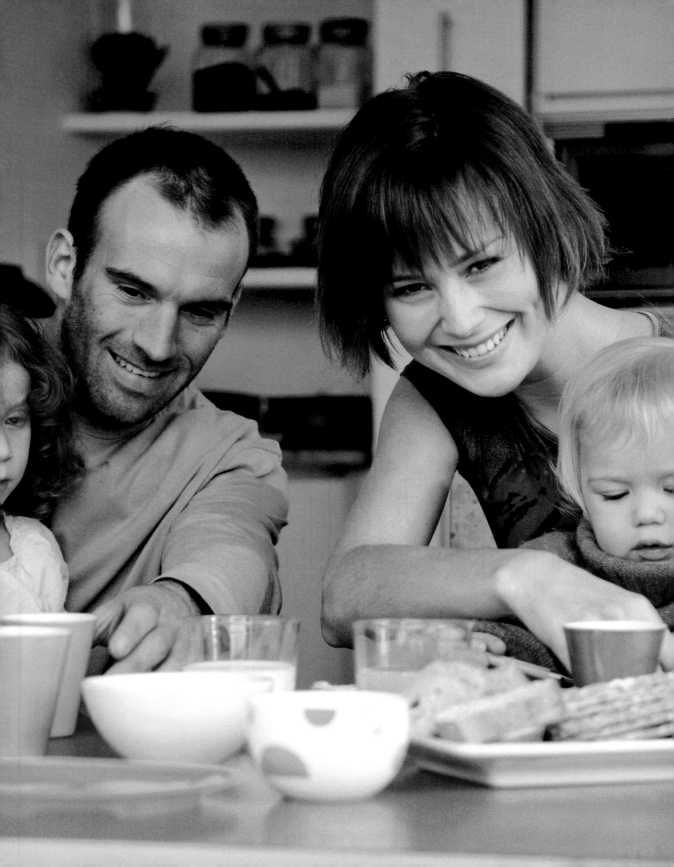

Oven-Baked Chicken Tenders

SERVES 4

2 cups Japanese-style panko bread crumbs

1 cup finely grated Parmesan cheese

3 tablespoons extra-virgin olive oil

Salt and freshly ground black pepper

2 tablespoons Dijon mustard

2 tablespoons mayonnaise

1 pound chicken tenders

1. Preheat the oven to 450°F. Fit a wire rack into a rimmed baking sheet.

2. Combine the panko, Parmesan, oil, and a pinch each of salt and pepper in a pie plate.

3. Combine the mustard and mayonnaise in a large bowl. Add the chicken tenders, tossing and turning until well coated. Then dredge the chicken in the panko until well coated. Transfer to the rack in a single layer.

4. Bake until golden brown and the meat loses its pinkness, about 12 minutes.

Chicken Tomato Quesadillas

SERVES 4

8 fajita-size flour tortillas (about 8 inches in diameter)

8 ounces Monterey Jack cheese, shredded

3 cups shredded cooked chicken

1 orange bell pepper, stemmed, seeded, and finely chopped

2 plum tomatoes, cored, seeded, and finely chopped

Sour cream, salsa, and lime wedges for serving, optional

1. Lightly grease, then heat an outdoor grill or grill pan over medium heat.

2. Lay the tortillas out. Sprinkle half of the cheese over the bottom halves of the tortillas. Top with the chicken, pepper, and tomatoes. Sprinkle the remaining cheese on top and fold the unfilled halves of the tortillas over the filled halves to form half-moons.

3. Carefully transfer the quesadillas to the grill in a single layer, working in batches if necessary. Cook until grill marks appear, about 3 minutes, then carefully turn each quesadilla over. Cook until grill marks appear and the cheese is melted, about 2 minutes.

4. Cool slightly, then cut into wedges.

Chicken Pot Pie

SERVES 8

Chicken

2 tablespoons extra-virgin olive oil

1¼ pounds skinless, boneless chicken breasts, cut into 1-inch chunks

Salt and freshly ground black pepper

1 large onion, finely chopped

2 medium carrots, cut into ½-inch chunks

1 medium celery root (celeriac), trimmed, peeled, and cut into ½-inch chunks

½ teaspoon fresh thyme leaves

1¾ cups low-sodium chicken broth

1½ cups whole milk

3 tablespoons cornstarch

1 cup frozen peas

Biscuit Topping

½ cup whole-wheat flour

½ cup all-purpose flour

1½ teaspoons baking powder

¼ teaspoon salt

1 teaspoon fresh thyme leaves, finely chopped

3 tablespoons butter

⅔ cup whole milk

1. Preheat the oven to 425°F.

2. To make the chicken: Heat 1 tablespoon oil in a large, deep ovenproof 12-inch skillet over high heat. Season the chicken with salt and pepper and add to the skillet in a single layer. Cook, turning the pieces over once, until golden, about 3 minutes. Transfer the chicken to a dish.

3. Heat the remaining oil in the skillet over medium heat. Add the onion, carrots, and celery root. Season with salt and pepper and cook, stirring occasionally, until the onion is tender, about 8 minutes. Add the thyme and cook, stirring, for 1 minute. Add the broth and bring to a boil.

4. Reduce the heat to maintain a steady simmer, cover, and cook until the carrots and

(CONTINUED)

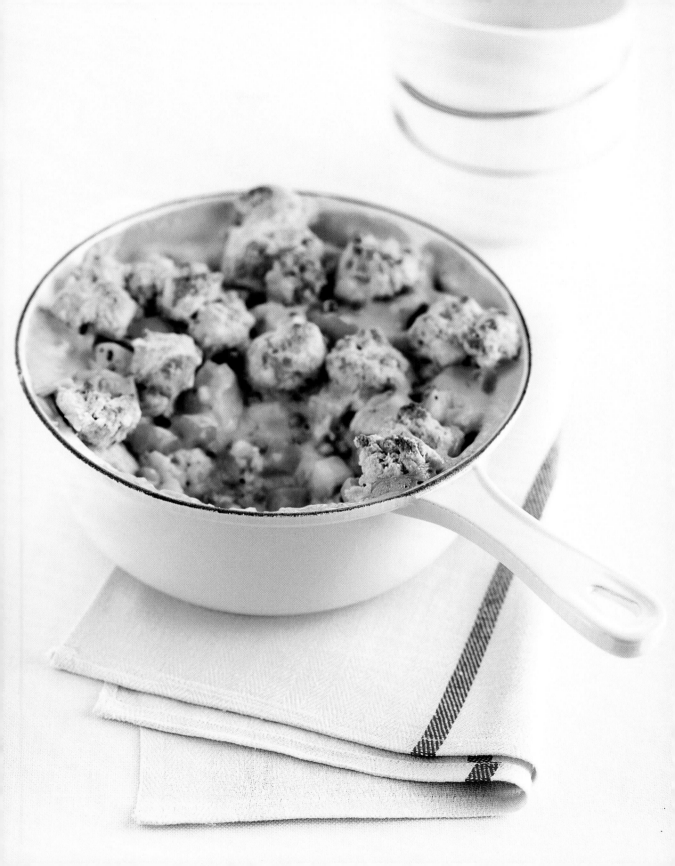

Chicken Pot Pie

(CONTINUED)

celery root are tender, about 10 minutes. Whisk together the milk and cornstarch until well combined. Stir into the mixture and cook for 2 minutes or until the sauce thickens. Stir in the peas and chicken and bring the mixture to a simmer, then remove from the heat.

5. Meanwhile, make the biscuit topping: Combine the flours, baking powder, salt, and thyme in a large bowl. With a pastry blender or your fingers, cut in the butter until coarse crumbs form. Stir in the milk just until the mixture comes together. Using a tablespoon, drop spoonfuls of the dough on top of the chicken mixture, spacing an inch apart. Transfer to the oven and bake 18 minutes or until the biscuits are golden brown and the chicken mixture is bubbling.

Spaghetti and Veggie Meat Sauce

SERVES 6

2 tablespoons extra-virgin olive oil

1 medium onion, finely chopped

2 carrots, finely chopped

2 red bell peppers, stemmed, seeded, and finely chopped

1 celery stalk, finely chopped

2 garlic cloves, finely chopped

Salt and freshly ground black pepper

1 pound ground turkey or lean ground beef

¼ teaspoon smoked paprika

1 (28-ounce) can crushed tomatoes in puree

1 tablespoon packed brown sugar

1 pound spaghetti

1. Heat the oil in a large, deep skillet over medium heat. Add the onion, carrots, peppers, celery, garlic, and a pinch each of salt and pepper. Cook, stirring occasionally, until the vegetables are tender, about 10 minutes.

2. Add the turkey and cook, stirring constantly and breaking up the meat, until the meat loses its pinkness, about 7 minutes. Stir in the paprika and cook, stirring, for 2 minutes.

3. Stir in the tomatoes and bring to a boil. Stir in the sugar, reduce the heat to medium-low, and simmer until thickened, about 30 minutes. (The sauce can be cooled and frozen at this point.)

4. Meanwhile, bring a large pot of water to a boil and salt it generously. Add the spaghetti and cook according to the package directions for al dente. Drain and return to the pot.

5. Add the pasta sauce to the spaghetti and cook, tossing constantly, over medium heat until well coated, about 2 minutes. Season to taste with salt and pepper.

Veggie Pizza

SERVES 4

1 cup chopped broccoli florets

1 pound fresh whole-wheat pizza dough

2½ cups shredded part-skim mozzarella cheese

1 yellow squash, diced

1 roasted red pepper, chopped

1 14.5-ounce can fire-roasted diced tomatoes, drained well

¼ cup freshly grated Parmesan cheese

1. Arrange an oven rack in the lowest position. Preheat the oven to 475°F.

2. Place the broccoli and 1 tablespoon water in a small microwave-safe bowl. Cover with plastic wrap and microwave on high until bright green and just tender, about 3 minutes. Drain well.

3. Pat, stretch, and shape the dough into a 14-inch round on a baking sheet. Scatter half of the mozzarella over the dough in an even layer, leaving a ½-inch rim. Scatter the squash, pepper, tomatoes, and broccoli over the cheese, then top with the Parmesan and remaining mozzarella.

4. Bake until the crust is golden brown and cooked through and the cheese melts, about 17 minutes. Cool slightly before slicing.

Fish Chowder

SERVES 4

2 bacon slices, chopped

1 medium onion, diced

1 medium celery root (celeriac), trimmed, peeled, and diced

1 pound red potatoes, diced

Salt and freshly ground black pepper

1 cup fish stock

2 cups corn kernels

2 cups whole milk

1 pound skinless salmon fillet, cut into 1-inch chunks

1 tablespoon snipped fresh chives

1. Place the bacon in a large saucepan and cook, stirring occasionally, over medium heat until crisp, about 5 minutes. Use a slotted spoon to transfer to paper towels to drain.

2. Add the onion, celery root, potatoes, and a pinch each of salt and pepper to the saucepan. Cook, stirring occasionally, until the onion is tender, about 7 minutes. Add the stock and bring to a boil over high heat. Stir in the corn, then reduce the heat to medium and simmer for 10 minutes.

3. Stir in the milk and continue simmering until the celery root and potatoes are tender, about 5 minutes. For a thicker chowder, mash some of the potatoes in the soup.

4. Gently stir in the salmon and simmer until the salmon just becomes opaque, about 3 minutes. Season to taste with salt and pepper. Garnish with chives and bacon.

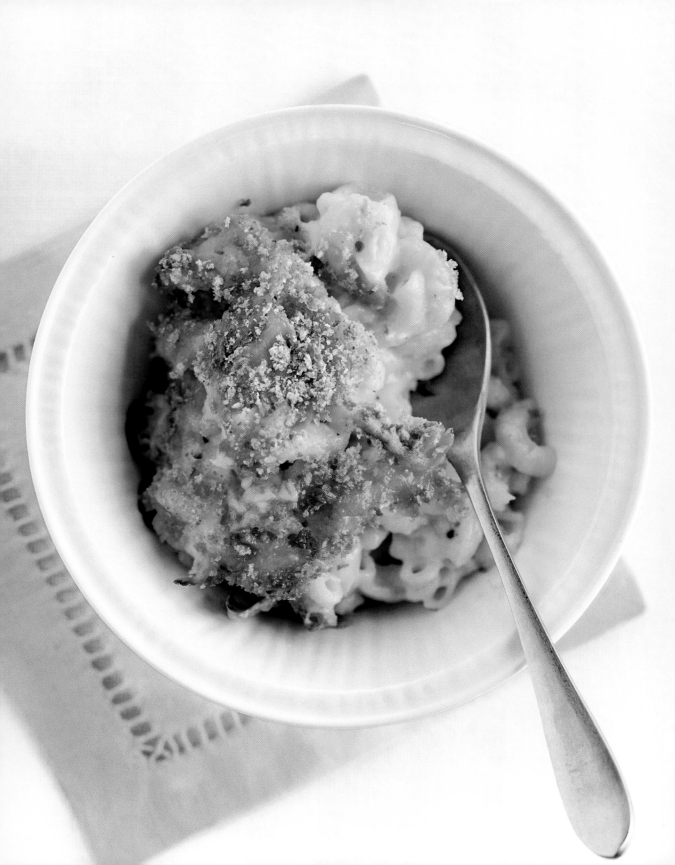

Homemade Mac and Cheese

SERVES 4

1 slice whole-wheat bread, torn into small pieces

3½ cups packed grated extra-sharp cheddar cheese

Salt and freshly ground black pepper

3 cups reduced-fat (2%) milk

4 tablespoons butter

¼ cup all-purpose flour

2½ cups small elbow macaroni

¼ teaspoon freshly grated nutmeg

1. Pulse the bread in a food processor to form fine crumbs. Transfer to a bowl and stir in ½ cup cheese and a pinch each of salt and pepper.

2. Arrange an oven rack 6 inches from the broiler heat source. Preheat the broiler.

3. Bring a large saucepan of salted water to a boil.

4. Microwave the milk on high for 4 minutes or until warm. Melt the butter in another large saucepan over medium heat. Add the flour and cook, whisking constantly, until mixture becomes pasty and golden, about 2 minutes. Continue whisking constantly while adding the milk in a slow, steady stream. Bring the mixture to a boil, whisking, then continue whisking for another 2 minutes.

5. Meanwhile, add the macaroni to the boiling water and cook until just tender, about 2 minutes less than the package's directions. Drain well.

6. Stir the remaining 3 cups cheese into the sauce, then stir in the macaroni and nutmeg. Season to taste with salt and pepper.

7. Transfer the mixture to a 2-quart baking dish and spread in an even layer. Top with an even layer of the crumbs. Broil just until golden brown on top, 1 to 2 minutes.

UFOs
(Unidentified Frying Objects)

SERVES 1

1 slice whole-grain sandwich bread

1 tablespoon butter, softened

1 large egg

Salt and freshly ground black pepper

1. Use a 3-inch round cookie cutter to cut a hole in the center of the bread. Spread half of the butter over one side of the bread slice and one side of the cut-out hole.

2. Melt the remaining butter in a medium skillet over medium heat. Add the bread and cut-out hole, buttered side up. Cook until golden brown on the bottom, about 1 minute, then turn over.

3. Break the egg into the hole in the bread. Season with a pinch of salt and pepper. Cook until the egg sets on the bottom and begins to set around the edges, about 2 minutes. Carefully flip the bread over and cook until the top of the egg is set, about 1 minute.

4. Serve with the cut-out hole for dunking into the egg center.

Waffles from La Leche League Baking Mix

MAKES 18

3 large eggs, separated

3 cups La Leche League Baking Mix (page 97)

2 cups whole milk

1. Preheat the oven to 200°F. Heat a waffle iron to medium. Grease if necessary.

2. In a large bowl, beat the egg whites until stiff, but not dry, peaks form.

3. In another large bowl, beat the yolks with the baking mix and milk until blended. Gently fold in the whites.

4. Pour batter into each waffle grid, adjusting the amount as necessary for your waffle iron model. Close and cook according to the waffle iron's manufacturer's directions until golden brown.

5. Transfer to a wire rack fitted into a rimmed baking sheet. Keep warm in the oven. Repeat with the remaining batter.

Pancakes from La Leche League Baking Mix

MAKES 18

3 cups La Leche League Baking Mix (page 97)

2 cups whole milk

2 large eggs, beaten

1. Heat a griddle or large cast iron or nonstick skillet over medium heat. Lightly grease if necessary.

2. Combine the baking mix, milk, and eggs in a large bowl. Stir until just blended.

3. Dollop large spoonfuls of batter onto the hot griddle to form 3-inch rounds. Cook until bubbles begin to form and pop on top, about 3 minutes. Flip and cook until golden brown on the bottom, about 2 minutes.

Smashed Potatoes

SERVES 4

1½ pounds small red potatoes (about 8), well scrubbed

Salt and freshly ground black pepper

½ cup reduced-fat (2%) milk

1 tablespoon butter

¼ cup sour cream

1. Place the potatoes in a large saucepan. Cover with cold water by 1 inch. Generously salt the water and bring to a boil over high heat. Reduce the heat to medium low, cover partially, and simmer until a knife pierces through very easily, about 30 minutes.

2. Combine the milk and butter in a microwave-safe measuring cup and microwave on high until very warm, about 1 minute.

3. Drain the potatoes and transfer to a large bowl. With a potato masher or fork, mash the potatoes until crushed. Add the sour cream and milk mixture and continue mashing until well combined. The potatoes should be mashed but still a little chunky. Season to taste with salt and pepper.

Roasted Beets with Balsamic Dressing

SERVES 4

6 medium beets (about 2 pounds), trimmed and scrubbed well

2 tablespoons extra-virgin olive oil

Salt and freshly ground black pepper

2 tablespoons balsamic vinegar

1. Preheat the oven to 425°F.

2. Wrap the beets in parchment paper, then wrap the parchment paper package tightly in foil. If the foil isn't tightly sealed, wrap with another layer of foil.

3. Place the beets on a rimmed baking sheet and roast until a knife pierces through easily, about 1 hour. Let stand in the packet until cool enough to handle, about 15 minutes. Peel the beets and cut into ½-inch chunks.

4. Transfer the beets to a large bowl, toss with the oil, and season with salt and pepper. Toss with the vinegar and serve.

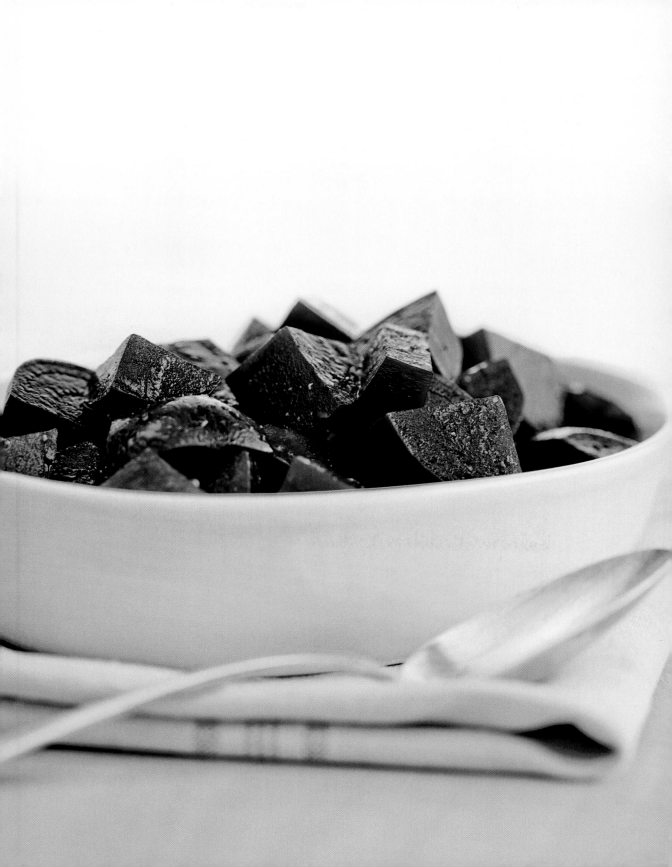

Sweet Potato Fries

SERVES 4

2 large sweet potatoes (about 1½ pounds)

½ teaspoon ground cumin

¼ teaspoon ground cinnamon

2 tablespoons canola oil

Salt and freshly ground black pepper

1. Preheat the oven to 425°F.

2. Peel the sweet potatoes, then cut each in half crosswise. Cut each half into 8 wedges lengthwise.

3. Toss the sweet potatoes with the cumin, cinnamon, oil, and a pinch each of salt and pepper in a large rimmed baking sheet until evenly coated. Spread in an even layer.

4. Bake, stirring once, until browned and tender, about 30 minutes.

Carrot-Zucchini Bread

MAKES 1 LOAF

1 cup all-purpose flour

1 cup whole-wheat flour

2 teaspoons baking powder

1 teaspoon ground allspice

½ teaspoon salt

1¼ cups sugar

1 cup canola oil

3 large eggs

¾ teaspoon vanilla extract

1 cup grated carrots

1 cup grated zucchini

½ teaspoon orange zest

¾ cup chopped walnuts, optional

1. Preheat the oven to 350°F. Lightly grease a 9-by-5-inch loaf pan.

2. Sift together the flours, baking powder, allspice, and salt in a large bowl.

3. Beat the sugar, oil, eggs, and vanilla in a medium bowl until well blended. Add to the flour mixture and stir until just combined. Fold in the carrots, zucchini, zest, and nuts. Transfer to the prepared pan.

4. Bake until a toothpick inserted in the center comes out clean, about 1 hour and 20 minutes.

5. Let cool in the pan on a wire rack for 20 minutes. Unmold and let cool completely on the wire rack.

One-Bowl Chocolate Cake

MAKES 1 (8-INCH) CAKE OR
1 DOZEN CUPCAKES

½ cup unsweetened cocoa powder

¾ cup all-purpose flour

¾ cup sugar

¾ teaspoon baking soda

½ teaspoon baking powder

¼ teaspoon salt

1 large egg

½ cup buttermilk

2 tablespoons canola oil

½ teaspoon pure vanilla extract

1. Preheat the oven to 350°F. If making a single cake, grease an 8-inch round cake pan, line the bottom with parchment paper, and grease again. If making cupcakes or mini cupcakes, line the tin with paper liners.

2. Whisk together the cocoa, flour, sugar, baking soda, baking powder, and salt in a large bowl. Add the egg, buttermilk, ⅓ cup warm water, oil, and vanilla and whisk until very smooth.

3. Pour the batter into the prepared pan or divide among the prepared cupcake cups.

4. Bake until a toothpick inserted in the center of the cake comes out clean, about 40 minutes for the cake, 20 minutes for the cupcakes, and 15 minutes for the mini cupcakes.

5. Let cool in the pan on a wire rack for 5 minutes, then remove from the pan and cool completely on the rack.

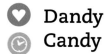

Dandy Candy

MAKES ABOUT 10 DOZEN

¼ cup nuts, finely chopped

½ cup finely shredded coconut

¼ cup sesame seeds

1 cup old-fashioned oats

1 cup dry milk powder

1 cup peanut butter

½ cup carob powder

½ cup honey

¼ cup wheat germ

1 teaspoon pure vanilla extract

1. Line a large rimmed baking sheet with wax paper. Combine the nuts, coconut, and sesame seeds on the pan and spread in an even layer.

2. Combine the oats, milk powder, peanut butter, carob powder, honey, wheat germ, 2 tablespoons water, and vanilla in a large bowl. Stir until very well mixed.

3. Scoop a rounded teaspoon of the mixture, roll into a ball, and place on the prepared pan. Repeat with the remaining mixture.

4. Gently roll the balls in the nut mixture until well coated, pressing to adhere. Cover and refrigerate for at least 1 hour and up to 1 week.

Dandy Candy: A Mother Remembers

My kids loved this recipe because it was so hands-on and no baking time, so it was quick. Their friends were always amazed how it tasted like chocolate without any chocolate in the recipe. My grown children still love this recipe and make it every now and then. This is a great recipe for kids to make.

—BARBARA

List of Recipes

The asterisks indicate La Leche League members' favorites.

Acknowledgments

We are grateful to the many dedicated and talented people who helped make this book possible.

Thank you!

- Writer Becky Cabaza: with twenty-five years' experience in the publishing industry, she seamlessly blended the philosophy found in our always popular cookbooks with updated recipes and nutrition information and did a wonderful job.
- Becky adds . . . Thanks to Stephanie Kip Rostan, who proved to be an astute matchmaker, and to Barbara Emanuel and LaJuana Oswalt for their wisdom, encouragement, and patience. Special thanks to Claire Dalidowitz for her vast knowledge of family nutrition and for her excellent sense of humor, to Genevieve Ko for her fabulous recipes, and to Marnie Cochran for her guidance and professionalism. Finally, thanks to my family for allowing me to work full steam (and monopolize our computer and Internet connection).
- Genevieve Ko: for the family-friendly, nutritious recipes. As senior food editor at Good Housekeeping Research Institute, Genevieve has contrib-

uted to other magazines including *Martha Stewart Living* and *Gourmet*. She has three little girls who are having fun learning their way around the kitchen.

- LLL Leader editors and reviewers: for their thoughtful and important review of the manuscript: ReNata Bauder, Barbara Emanuel, Kathy Grossman, Barbara Higham, Diana Lewis, LaJuana Oswalt, Shirley Phillips, and Diana West.
- Stephanie Kip-Rostan: our friend and literary agent at Levine Greenberg for her valuable guidance, expertise, and unending patience.
- Senior Editor Marnie Cochran: who guided and trusted us on this project, and the great team at Random House for all their help in bringing this project together.
- A very special photographer: Katrine Naleid; food stylist Jen Straus; and prop stylist Jaimi Holker for luscious photos that are truly magical.
- The LLLI office staff: for their creative ideas and contributions on this project: Barbara, Dave, Holly, Jackie, LaJuana, Nicole, Ron, Sandhya, and Susan.
- . . . and most important, to the Leaders and families who have contributed to and supported La Leche League International around the world as we celebrate fifty-five years of helping mothers and babies.

Conversion Charts

GAS MARK	FAHRENHEIT	CELSIUS	DESCRIPTION
¼	225	110	very cool / very slow
½	250	130	---
1	275	140	cool
2	300	150	---
3	325	170	very moderate
4	350	180	moderate
5	375	190	---
6	400	200	moderately hot
7	425	220	hot
8	450	230	---
9	475	240	very hot

LARGE VOLUME EQUIVALENTS

1 cup	8 fluid ounces	½ pint	
2 cups	16 fluid ounces	1 pint	
3 cups	24 fluid ounces	1-½ pints	¾ quart
4 cups	32 fluid ounces	2 pints	1 quart
6 cups	48 fluid ounces	3 pints	1-½ quarts
8 cups	64 fluid ounces	2 quarts	½ gallon
16 cups	128 fluid ounces	4 quarts	1 gallon

SMALL VOLUME EQUIVALENTS

1 tablespoon	3 teaspoons	$\frac{1}{2}$ fluid ounce
2 tablespoons	$\frac{1}{8}$ cup	1 fluid ounce
4 tablespoons	$\frac{1}{4}$ cup	2 fluid ounces
5 tablespoons	$\frac{1}{3}$ cup	2-$\frac{1}{3}$ fluid ounces + 1 tsp
6 tablespoons	$\frac{3}{8}$ cup	3 fluid ounces
8 tablespoons	$\frac{1}{2}$ cup	4 fluid ounces
10 tablespoons	$\frac{2}{3}$ cup	5-$\frac{1}{3}$ fluid ounces + 2 tsp
12 tablespoons	$\frac{3}{4}$ cup	6 fluid ounces
14 tablespoons	$\frac{7}{8}$ cup	7 fluid ounces
16 tablespoons	1 cup	8 fluid ounces

METRIC CONVERSION CHART

1 teaspoon	5 ml
1 tablespoon	15 ml
$\frac{1}{4}$ cup	60 ml
$\frac{1}{3}$ cup	80 ml
$\frac{1}{2}$ cup	120 ml
$\frac{2}{3}$ cup	160 ml
$\frac{3}{4}$ cup	180 ml
1 cup	240 ml
1 pint	475 ml
1 quart	.95 liter
1 gallon	3.8 liters

Notes

CHAPTER 1

1. According to the American Congress of Obstetricians and Gynecologists (ACOG), "moderate" caffeine consumption of 200 milligrams per day, the amount in about two 8-ounce cups of brewed coffee, "does not appear to lead to miscarriage or preterm birth." Check with your health care provider for more information and view ACOG's recommendations at www.acog.org/publications/patient_education/bp001.cfm.

2. Developed by Claire K. Dalidowitz, M.S., M.A., R.D., CD-N (certified dietitian-nutritionist), clinical nutrition services manager at Connecticut Children's Medical Center.

CHAPTER 2

1. The reference/recommended daily intakes (RDI) of nutrients used in this book are based on standards set by the United States Food and Drug Administration.

2. Nancy Mohrbacher and Julie Stock, *The Breastfeeding Answer Book,* 3rd ed. (Schaumburg, IL: La Leche League International, 2003, 436).

3. The nutritional information on fruits and vegetables is from www.fruitsandveggiesmorematters.org, sponsored by the nonprofit consumer education and public health organization Produce for Better Health Foundation in conjunction with the U.S. government.

4. If you'd like to read more about this topic, start with the work of Walter J. Rogan, M.D., a preeminent specialist in pediatric epidemiology who has published and initiated major studies in this area.

5. You may wish to choose a plastic water bottle labeled as "BPA-free." Bisphenol A (BPA) is a chemical used in the production of plastic bottles and reusable plastic containers, as well as in plastic liners of canned goods. Though there are no studies on human ingestion of BPA, high doses of BPA have caused harm in lab animals. It is easier to find BPA-free products such as water bottles as manufacturers have responded to consumer demand.

6. From *New Beginnings* (published by La Leche League International), Vol. 23, No. 5 (September–October 2006): 220–21.

CHAPTER 3

1. Excerpted from Inbal Bahar, "Eating Wisely by Exchanging Food with Your Friends on a Regular Basis," *New Beginnings*, Vol. 2, No. 1 (2009), © La Leche League International, Inc.

2. As reported in Gina Kolata, "Doubt Is Cast on Many Reports of Food Allergies," *New York Times*, May 11, 2010. Dr. Marc Reidl, an allergist and immunologist, published his findings based on food allergy versus food intolerance in the May 12, 2010, issue of the *Journal of the American Medical Association*, "Diagnosing and Managing Common Food Allergies: A Systematic Review." According to its conclusion: "The evidence for the prevalence and management of food allergy is greatly limited by a lack of uniformity for criteria for making a diagnosis."

3. "One long-term study of children who were breastfed showed that breastfeeding reduces food allergies at least through adolescence (Grasky 1982). Protection from allergies is one of the most important benefits of breastfeeding. The incidence of cow's milk allergies is up to seven times greater in babies who are fed artificial baby milk instead of human milk (Lawrence 1994)." From Karen Zeretzke, "Allergies and the Breastfeeding Family," *New Beginnings*, Vol. 15, No. 4 (July–August 1998): 100, © La Leche League International, Inc.

CHAPTER 4

1. According to a statement from the American Heart Association, "The majority (up to 75 percent) of sodium that Americans consume comes from sodium added to processed foods by manufacturers. While some of this sodium is added to foods for safety reasons—the amount of salt added to processed foods is clearly above and beyond what is required for safety and function of the food supply." www.americanheart.org/presenter.jhtml?identifier=4708.

2. Margaret Kenda, *Whole Foods for Babies and Toddlers* (Schaumburg, IL: La Leche League International, 2001).

3. These are FDA-approved terms, found at www.americanheart.org/presenter.jhtml ?identifier=4708. For more information on sodium and other ingredient labeling, see the nutrition labeling definitions at www.fda.gov/Food/GuidanceComplianceRegulatoryInformation/ GuidanceDocuments/FoodLabelingNutrition/FoodLabelingGuide/ucm064911.htm.

4. As quoted in Laura Flynn McCarthy, "Baby's First Foods," Parenting.com, www.parenting.com/article/babys-first-foods-starting-solids?page=0,7.

5. For more information, see www.baby-led.com and the related book by Gill Rapley and Tracey Murkett, *Baby-Led Weaning: Helping Your Baby to Love Good Food* (London: Vermilion, 2008).

CHAPTER 5

1. Available for purchase on our website at www.llli.org.

2. From Margaret Kenda, *Whole Foods for Babies and Toddlers* (Schaumburg, IL: La Leche League International, 2001). These guidelines are also consistent with recommendations from the AAP.

Index

Photo Credits

Would You Like to Know More?

La Leche League International (LLLI) is a source of information, support, and encouragement. La Leche League groups meet all over the world to share breastfeeding and mothering experiences. To become a member of LLLI, find your local group, or Leader in your community, or for more LLLI information, visit the LLLI website at llli.org.

La Leche League International offers many resources in addition to our new 8th edition of *The Womanly Art of Breastfeeding*, which is a national bestseller. llli.org/thewomanlyartofbreastfeeding

Local Resources

- Accredited La Leche League Leaders are available in seventy countries:llli.org/webindex.html
- Gatherings of mothers, babies, and LLLI Leaders for information and support
- Phone and online help from accredited LLLI Leaders

Online Support and Information

- Mother-to-mother forums: forums.llli.org
- Help forms (mothers enter questions online and receive personalized answers from La Leche League Leaders via email): llli.org/help_form
- Breastfeeding answers on a variety of topics of interest—general breastfeeding, maternal breastfeeding, infant/child breastfeeding, families, nutrition, and more
- Social media sites such as Facebook: tinyrul.com/lllifacebook and Twitter: tinyurl.com/lllitwitter

Online support can be accessed by clicking the "Resources" link on our website homepage at llli.org or go to llli.org/resources.html

Publications

- Books on a variety of subjects and languages such as breastfeeding, parenting, nutrition, children's books, and professional texts
- Information sheets—*breastfeeding tips, is my baby getting enough milk?, establishing your milk supply*—for a full listing of LLLI products visit: store.llli.org
- Online e-magazines, updates, and special announcements: llli.org/breastfeedingtoday

Our printed publications are available in our online store at store.llli.org or directly from our home page via the navigational tab. Additional publications are offered to members by various LLL entities around the world. These can be found by visiting the local websites linked on the llli.org home page.